To Mona,
with love

A Peruvian Psychiatric Hospital

William W. Stein

University Press of America, Inc.
Lanham • New York • London

4720 Boston Way
Lanham, Maryland 20706

3 Henrietta Street
London, WC2E 8LU England

Printed in the United States of America
British Cataloging in Publication Information Available

Library of Congress Cataloging-in-Publication Data

Stein, William W.
A Peruvian psychiatric hospital / William W. Stein.
p. cm.
Includes bibliographical references and index.
1. Psychiatric hospitals--Peru--Sociological aspects. 2. Psychiatric hospital care--Peru. 3. Hospital Víctor Larco Herrera (Lima, Peru)--History. I. Title.
(DNLM: 1. Hospitals, Psychiatric--Peru. 2. Mental Disorders--therapy. WM 28 DP6 S8p 1995)
RC451.P4S74 1995 362.2'1'098525 --dc20 95-35758 CIP
DNLM/DLC
for Library of Congress

ISBN 0-7618-0093-X (cloth: alk: ppr.)

The paper used in this publication meets the minimum requirements of American National Standard for Information Sciences—Permanence of Paper for Printed Library Materials, ANSI Z39.48—1984

Contents

Foreword

by Javier Mariátegui, M.D.

I am a privileged witness to the process of this book's gestation. I knew William W. Stein when, supported by a Fulbright Grant, he came to Peru in 1959 with the double purpose of occupying the Chair of Social Anthropology in the Faculty of Letters of the University of San Marcos and of doing research in the field of social psychiatry, at that time with its greatest popularity, employing the techniques of interviewing and participant observation.

Stein made Pavilion 20 of the Hospital Víctor Larco Herrera, in Magdalena del Mar, a part of the city of Lima, the privileged site of his research. This pavilion was of recent construction (having been opened in 1957) but a part of an old hospital, the building of which had begun at the end of the last century. The facility was put to psychiatric use only in 1918, to replace the Hospicio del Cercado (Inner City Hospice, also referred to as "Insane Asylum") which was Peru's first psychiatric institution. The Hospital Víctor Larco Herrera for years had been called the Asilo-Colonia de la Magdalena (Asylum Plantation of La Magdalena) in order to indicate its character of offering shelter and rehabilitating patients through agricultural work. It changed its name from asylum to hospital in 1930 with the new administration of its second Director, Dr. Baltazar Caravedo Prado. At that time the

Hospital was controlled by the Public Charity Society of Lima. It was transferred to the public sector in 1967 when the Ministry of Health took over.

Pavilion 20 was in 1959 the most active of all the services for charity patients in the Hospital both from its recent and modern construction and from its character as the instructional site of the Professorate of Psychiatry of the University of San Marcos. Although two psychiatrists were appointed to head this unit, there were more than ten others of us who labored there on different schedules and were "unripe psychiatrists," as the Director, Dr. Juan Francisco Valega, liked to call us, that is, "green" psychiatrists in the process of maturation.[1] A few of us came every day, including Sundays and holidays. Those were the times of new drugs for the treatment of mental illnesses, so that several substances, especially neuroleptics and antidepressants, were tried out in the Hospital, notably in Pavilion 20, with both inpatients and outpatients. The first observations with thioridacine (Melleril), imipramine (Tofranil), and amitriptiline (Tryptanol) were made in this service, which called for very close following of the subjects, daily for inpatients and weekly for ambulatory patients. In Pavilion 20 we lived through a period of intense and modernized attendance in accord with the rhythm of the times. It was the "boom" of social psychiatry and the acme of the psychopharmacological era. Meanwhile, other Hospital pavilions retained the character of old custodial institutions, madhouses.

The free time which the teaching of his course in San Marcos allowed him Stein dedicated to the Hospital, the mornings in Pavilion 20 and the afternoons in the other services, including those for paying-patients. He interviewed patients, psychiatrists, nurses, social workers, attendants, and so on. His basic knowledge of Quechua, the principal aboriginal Peruvian language, permitted the breaking of the wall of resistance which Andean mestizo populations have in relation to the "gringo," especially the "yanqui." Stein studied the interactions among the different levels of staff with patients, and of patients among themselves. He took notes naturally and avoided the suspicion of the recorded voice that exists among us ("whoever carries off my recorded voice, carries off something of myself, of my privacy," is something that any one of his interview subjects could have said).

Some of Stein's experiences in the psychiatric hospital were written as articles abroad and published in English in anthropological and social psychiatric journals.[2] Therefore, the book we now have available has been preceeded by those publications. In spite of the time that has passed between the original observations and now, the data which appear here offer a total image which is not only of historical interest but also of practical utility, which should be taken into account in the organization of psychiatric establishments today, a time when the big asylums have declined completely. Now, thanks to communitarian and social techniques, and to neuroleptics, care can be offered to patients without breaking their family and other social relations, and their recuperation can be accelerated.[3]

A Peruvian Psychiatric Hospital brings together the several aspects of the psychiatric institution seen from a social anthropological perspective. The first Chapter takes up "Images of Peruvian Psychiatry" with statements from the physicians of different pavilions in the Hospital Víctor Larco Herrera. In Chapter 2, one of the richest, Stein analyzes concepts of mental illness as expressed by patients, psychiatrists, psychologists, nurses, and attendants. Prevailing ideologies are examined, ideas that range from the most evolved conceptions of mental illness of professional persons, impregnated with Eurocentric scientific psychiatry, to the notions of mental health workers which contain remnants of traditional medicine and the evaluations and prejudices of aboriginal cultures and national society in transition.

Chapter 3 asks, "What is a Mental Hospital?" and implies "what is a mental hospital in Peru?" It examines the responses of the personnel who serve in it. Here, as in the earlier chapters, appears the invariable presence of the theoretical model which orients Stein's essays from his readings in sociology and other pertinent branches of the study of human behavior, which he extracts from both world and Peruvian literature. Chapter 4, "Being a Mental Patient in Peru, presents the opinions of mental patients about the nature of the illness, conditioning factors, and the changes taking place in them as they respond to life in the pavilion. An appendix presents a list of the interview subjects and their diagnoses.

Chapter 5 examines the social roles that are performed in the interaction of the several strata of caretaking personnel with each other and with patients. Deficiencies in the organization of work appear in each professional, technical, or service stratum, which thinks and acts more in conformity with its own conceptions than those inculcated by the Institution. The social roles place in relief a certain autonomy among the caregivers, as if, in the search for their own functions, they do not grasp their performance in relation to the others. The fragmentary character of the resulting labor is a reflection as much of the expectations of Peruvian society as of the defensive deformation of roles produced by work that demands at one and the same time subtlety in interpersonal engagement and a reaffirmation of the "principle of authority" as a means of personal reassurance for the management of large groups of patients.

Chapter 6 is devoted to the attendants, modest representatives of the popular sector, to whom are assigned tasks of little or no splendor, but a stratum which consists of people who are physically and culturally closest to the daily lives of the patients of a psychiatric hospital. It is a group with "deferred hopes," aware of its subordination, subject to the criticism of the physicians and nurses, almost always misunderstood, and rarely appreciated. There is in the presentation of this group of attendants an empathetic drawing close on the part of the book's author much appreciated by those of us who approach this postponed sector with social sensitivity in our evaluation of the social dynamics of psychiatric care.

Chapter 7 is centered on the nurses, the profession of "mistaken identities," as the author calls it. There exists a Nursing Supervisors' office in the Hospital, but in practice nurses depend directly on the doctors. They carry out many of the functions of the latter by delegation or because these functions must be peformed by someone in the Hospital's strict line of authority. In psychiatry, the nurse's labor is more complex than in general hospital practice. Nurses carry out polyvalent roles and they must engage in, in addition to the classic functions of the dispensary, an intense relation with the patients, their relatives, and the entire personnel of the hospital. This professional sector should be close to patients and devote the greatest time to them, but they are wage-earners who need second jobs as private nurses for patients with economic resources or in other psychiatric services.

William W. Stein's interest in the native population of Peru began in the early 1950s when he conducted research in the community of Hualcán, located in the Province of Carhuaz in the Department of Ancash. His Cornell University doctoral thesis of 1955 was later published as a book (*Hualcan: Life in the Highlands of Peru.* Ithaca, New York: Cornell University Press, 1961). Later he worked in Vicos, a few miles south of Hualcán, the site of the Peru-Cornell Project, a cooperative research effort on an international scale by the Instituto

Indigenista del Perú and Cornell University. His long academic career did not interfere with the maintenance of his frequent and active ties with Peru, especially with the highlands of the Department of Ancash. As the culmination of his academic activity, Stein is today Professor Emeritus in the Department of Anthropology, State University of New York at Buffalo.

He has published several other books on Peru: *El levantamiento de Atusparia, el movimiento popular ancashino de 1885* (Lima: Mosca Azul Editores, 1988); *Mariátegui y Norka Rouskaya, crónica de la presunta profanación del Cementerio de Lima en 1917* (Lima: Empresa Editora Amauta, 1989); and *Los becerros hambrientos y otros ensayos de antropología económica peruana* (Lima: Mosca Azul Editores, 1991). He has also edited a book in North America (*Peruvian Contexts of Change* (New Brunswick, New Jersey: Transaction Books, 1985), and published several chapters in it and other books on Peruvian reality, as well as a number of journal articles. Included in his works are essays on traditional Peruvian medicine and psychiatric sociology.

Stein is a truly exceptional person, with diverse talents, cordial and warm, who spontaneously establishes empathetic relations with other persons, and who has great social sensitivity, especially with aboriginal populations. He has shed light on a good part of anthropological knowledge in contemporary Peru. He is an authentic Peruvianist and has been an excellent personal friend for more than three decades, all of which gives me great pleasure in writing this Preface to the English edition of *A Peruvian Psychiatric Hospital.*

Javier Mariátegui, M.D., Ph.D.
Titular Member of the National Academy of Medicine
Titular Member of the Peruvian Academy of Language
Professor Emeritus, University of San Marcos
Principal Professor of the Honorio Delgado Chair, Cayetano Heredia University

Notes

1. The Head Physician of Pavilion 20 was at that time Professor Honorio Delgado, a great figure in Spanish-language psychiatry of the present century, who was Principal Professor in what was at that time the only Faculty of Medicine existing in the country, in the University of San Marcos, and who held the same position in other services of the Hospital (Pavilions 2, 8, and 18). He delegated responsibility for the operation of Pavilion 20 to the two Assistant Physicians, Drs. Alfredo Saavedra Villalobos and Pedro Aliaga Lindo.

2. Stein (1963a, 1963b, 1993a, 1993b), Stein and Oetting (1964), Oetting and Stein (1966).

3. The first neuroleptic drug to be used in Peru was tried out in Pavilion 20. See Mariátegui, et al. (1966).

Acknowledgments

The original research was carried out while I was in Peru in 1959 as Fulbright Lecturer in Social Anthropology in the University of San Marcos. My thanks are due to the Peruvian Fulbright Commission for its assistance in initiating the project. Drs. Baltazar Caravedo Caranza and Javier Mariátegui were also instrumental in getting the project going, the first for introducing me to the Hospital, and the second for bringing me to Pavilion 20. The late Dr. Humberto Rotondo took a helpful interest in the research; his kindness will not be forgotten. Dr. Mariátegui has remained a constant friend and generous host during thirty years. Analysis of the data began in 1960 with the assistance of a Small Grant (M-4371[A]) from the National Institute of Mental Health. Without the kindness and goodwill of the personnel and patients of the Hospital Víctor Larco Herrera the research would have been impossible; I am profoundly grateful to them. I also want to express my appreciation of the help given to me by my friend and colleague in the Department of Anthropology, State University of New York at Buffalo, Donald Pollock, who shared enthusiastically his personal library and pointed out a path. Zoe Zacharek has read the manuscript and made many helpful suggestions for improving the style, but she has had nothing to do with its defects. I also thank State University of Buffalo's Computinmg Center and its consultants, without whose assistance this book never would have taken shape. My children,

Dan and Sue, who are also my best teachers, are ever sources of love and inspiration, and I thank them for their support.

Unless otherwise indicated, all translations from the Spanish are my own.

This book is being published simultaneously in a Spanish edition by Mosca Azul Editores, Lima.

I thank Renato D. Alarcón for permission to reproduce in English translation materials from his publication, Renato D. Alarcón, ed., *Identidad de la psiquiatría latinoamericana* (Mexico City: Siglo Veintiuno Editores, 1990).

W.W.S.

Chapter 1

Images of Peruvian Psychiatry

I select for presentation here one portion of the research materials, from my study in 1959 of the Hospital Víctor Larco Herrera in Lima, Peru, which relates to the images psychiatrists projected of their professional lives and selves. Although I acknowledge the constraints time imposes on me, in the sense that I am dealing with conditions of a period that is now a generation ago, many of those conditions have persisted into the present particularly in regard to the Hospital's understaffed, underbudgeted, and overpopulated charity services. It is my hope to write not simply a historical chronicle of this sector of a larger hospital world but, more ambitiously, to tell Peruvians, and more particularly Peruvian psychiatrists, some things about themselves they may not have known, things that may be of some help in planning for a better future.

The study was conducted between August 12 and December 24, 1959 mainly, but not exclusively, in Pavilion 20, a charity unit (designated in Spanish as *régimen común*, or "ordinary treatment") that serviced an in-patient population which averaged around seventy men, eighty per cent of whom were diagnosed as schizophrenic, the rest being manic-depressive, alcoholic, epileptic, and other categories; and about three hundred out-patients with a similar diagnostic profile. As of December 4, there was a total of 1248 patients in the hospital, 694 males and 554 females, divided into 300 paying patients, which included many covered by insurance, and 948 charity patients. The staff consisted of 47 medical personnel, 82 certified nurses (graduates of the School of Nursing on the hospital grounds), 448 workers who were classfied as "laborers" for social security purposes, and 43 administrative personnel, classified as "employees" for another social security system. The hospital consisted of twenty pavilions, differentiated according to sex, age, varying mixes of chronic and acute diagnoses, medical complications (i.e., internal medicine and tuberculosis), legal status, new admissions, and the variety of dietary plans ("extras," "first," "second," "third," and "charity") pivoting on the amount and quality of food and the availability of medications. In addition there was a nursing home and a "labor therapy" shop which earned profits for the administration. Inside the Hospital grounds there was also a Nursing School, offering a standard three-year course, which produced psychiatric nurses; at the time, it contained 56 students who lived on the premises.

The physicians, who are identified by pseudonyms in this essay, were divided into chiefs of service (4), assistant physicians with stipends (35), free assistants without stipends (8), comparable to senior residents, and a continually changing number of voluntary assistants comparable to junior residents, also without stipends, who were acquiring clinical experience. These doctors were distributed among the pavilions according to the graded dietary categories: thus, one with 22 paying patients could have 4 doctors while another with 233 charity patients could have 2. The Hospital usually assigned 2 nurses to each pavilion, one for the day and another at night, but if the patient population was more than 50 this assignment could be doubled. Additional nurses were also assigned for specialized treatments. The pavilions were also assigned from 7 to 26 attendants each.

In Pavilion 20, the chief physician appeared briefly once or twice a week, early in the morning; the two assistant physicians kept fairly regular schedules; the one free assistant appeared daily for several hours (he was there so often and was so active that when I first began my observations in the pavilion I imagined he was the chief); and two of the four voluntary assistants appeared to spend more time there, while the other two were there less frequently. With the exception of the chief, a psychiatrist who was highly regarded by his colleagues, nationally and internationally, and whom I did not get to know well because he had his primary responsibilities in another pavilion, all these staff persons, as well as several others I came to know in other pavilions, demonstrated a high degree of personal involvement in what they were doing, commitment to their profession, and frustration by the limitations imposed by hospital realities, in the sense of restrictions on what they felt they could accomplish in the context of the structure of the hospital and the scant resources available to them.

The poverty of the Hospital reflected the general poverty prevailing in Peru, an underdeveloped country, a circumstance that makes psychiatric practice quite a different and a much more difficult experience from comparable professional activity in a developed country. Alarcón (1990:30-31), a Peruvian psychiatrist, comments on this challenge in Latin America as a whole:

> Subject to pressures and demands of the most varied nature, on our continent, the psychiatrist's being and activity, as well as those of his profession, confront the distressing weight of ambiguity, if not the painful sting of impotence. Neither the one nor the other are necessarily or uniquely his responsibility. . . . The psychiatrist can not, he should not, and, happily, he is not alien to his circumstances. As long as it is not understood that mental health constitutes the root and essence of complete health, the psychiatrist will continue to see tiny amounts of the national budget devoted to his specialty. He will also continue to see discouragement, demoralization, and fury enter the collective spirit with the same or greater brutality as the bacillus enters the lungs of its victims. And he will likewise observe the growing erosion of the principles of solidarity and respect for human dignity, weakening if not corroding a weak and unpredictable political apparatus.
>
> And the psychiatrist has to live. . . . So it happens that the average psychiatrist . . . serves a relatively small sector of the population--thanks to which, nevertheless, he and his family survive--at the same time that he is clearly and sadly conscious that enormous masses of human beings have no opportunity whatsoever to benefit from his assistance. It will be said that this is the reality for all professional physicians in Latin America. However, it is clear that for the psychiatrist, more than for any other medical specialist, this tragic paradox acquires particularly cruel dimensions: by vocation, by formation, by daily activity, by nature, we feel more intensely the outcry at inequality and the anguish of its victims.
>
> To be a psychiatrist and to do psychiatry . . . is a challenge to the very core of what we call professional identity. It is a continual

> challenge to the moral integrity of its cultivators. It is a struggle raised by the conflicts which confront affluence, comfort, and prestige on one side, with the moral urgencies of a lacerating reality on the other. Being a psychiatrist . . . puts to the test a presence of spirit, a tolerance for frustration, flexibility, and adaptability to a world in explainable but uninteligible effervescence.

In 1959, the Hospital Víctor Larco Herrera was the only separate psychiatric facility in Peru, although two other general hospitals, facilities provided by Peru's two social security systems, the Obrero (for laborers) and the Empleado (for employees), had twenty psychiatric beds each. The postgraduate physician who wished to specialize in psychiatry, therefore, was extremely limited in the selection of his or her training site. This was unfortunate because the political nature of the hospital, an appendage of the Lima Public Charity Society,[1] intensified many of the human weaknesses of its personnel. I recorded these passages in my observational notes of conversations with Dr. Lleras:

> Dr. Lleras and I talked about organizational structure, the work load, and administrative problems. He said the administration puts pressure on the doctors. The administrators are budget conscious and want things to look good at the end of the year. . . . They hired two new secretaries recently but will not give doctors what they need. They have canceled subscriptions to psychiatric journals and do not add books to the library any more.
>
> Dr. Lleras says the administration is too budget conscious. There are too many clerks and secretaries in the administration and not enough workers and nurses in the pavilions. . . . It is hard for a charity patient to get in the hospital unless he can get someone in the administration or the Charity Society to help. The aim of the hospital is to make a profit. Occupational therapy is a joke because profits are made by the Supervisor of Nursing and the Administrator. He gets over three thousand soles [at about 27 soles to the dollar in 1959] a month, plus food, housing, servants, use of a car, and so on.
>
> Dr. Lleras says that the Director has very little power; he is a shadow. One of the doctors belongs to the managing committee of the Charity Society and the Director does not. This makes for an impossible situation. Then, the Administrator really runs the place and can have anything he wants. Politics has a great deal to do with the admission of patients, if people have no money. The Administrator lets in anybody he wants; that is how patronage enters

> into the hospital. Many acute outpatients need hospital treatment but have to be taken care of at home, which puts pressure on the family, especially if the rest of them have to earn a living.

In answer to the question, "In which pavilions have you worked and which do you prefer?", Dr. Díaz responded:

> Pavilions x__, y__ and z__. I prefer none of them. They are all the same filth, because nothing is done for the patients. They ought to set off an atomic bomb and blow it all up, the pavilions and the people. And then begin again. I love my chief of service, but he can't do anything either. The chiefs are all different. Some are able to get things, but then they use them to reinforce their own prestige.

However, the greatest problem the doctors faced was not the hospital's poverty but, rather, their own.[2] This report of a conversation with Dr. Méndez, whose primary affiliation was with another hospital, begins to describe these circumstances:

> Dr. Méndez said the doctors at his hospital are better off with regard to salary. He himself has no economic worries because his father is comfortably well off. However, the salary is good. In contrast, Larco Herrera pays a miserable salary. Dr. Noriega is well off, but Dr. Méndez knows doctors who must try to subsist on the salary, which is not enough. Many of them have to take outside jobs, doing all kinds of things that are not medical. Consequently, they have no time to study, and a person is lost if he cannot keep up with the reading. Dr. Méndez said I should look at the doctors' homes. Some of them live only a step above medical students, who often live four in a small room.

Most of the doctors appeared always to be in a hurry. They expressed a concern with time and the necessity of dividing it among the various subsistence occupations that appear to make up what I have called a "laminated livelihood" (Stein 1984:286), and what Peruvians refer to as "the seven trades and fourteen needs" of poor people who have to construct a living as best they can. It is characteristic of peasants in the hinterland but it applies equally well to Peruvian professional medical persons.[3] With the exception of a few, like Dr. Méndez, the doctors tried to put a living together by working in a variety of other hospitals and clinics, as well as in their own private practice, on the para-medical margins as medical publishers' representatives and pharmaceutical salesmen, and outside medicine as accountants and school teachers. Here are some of my observations on the theme:

> Dr. Ñique says he comes here every day but he has a job at a high school that makes him two hours late on Mondays and Wednesdays. He gets S/.1,300 [something over $46. at the time] a month for it. It is very little but it helps because the pay here is very low. He says he has private practice in the afternoons. He has a few patients for therapy, but he mostly handles referrals from other doctors. He specializes and there are only a few others in Lima who can do what he does.
>
> Dr. Alba says he has a headache and goes to the sink where he draws water and gulps down a pink pill. He says the morning goes too fast. He has to go to his private practice which he has on three afternoons a week. On the other three afternoons he prepares lectures for one class of medical students and another for psychology students. Then he also works on the mental hygiene study of the shantytowns. He has no time!
>
> Dr. Caso asks me how the morning seemed to me. I answer, busier than usual. I ask him how many jobs he has. He answers, on Tuesdays interviewing patients here; he has twelve and is required to write reports on them once a week. On Thursdays, he has a class for nurses here, and then the conference on cases with Dr. Fernández. On other days he works in a general hospital with an outpatient clinic, and teaches a course for nurses at another general hospital. In the afternoons he has his private patients. He says he takes five minutes for lunch, sometimes naps, but usually just goes on working.

Extracts from the interview questions on occupational history amplify these observations:

> Dr. Bueno: I'm an assistant physician here. They pay me S/.850 a month. I also work as a primary school teacher in the District of X_____. I'm in charge of one section of second grade with fifty pupils. I work from 1:30 to 5:15 on Monday to Saturday. Actually, we work from 2 to 5. Later I work in the evening in the District of Y_____, in night school from 7 to 10. It's fifth grade. I also work in the Department of Mental Hygiene, in the research department.

I'm a member of a team. Then I have my office hours from 5 to 7 every day. I work generally by appointment. I take in S/.8,000 monthly, all together. The biggest part is from teaching, S/.5,000. I had left teaching to work as a professional, but my friends advised me to return so I would complete my service years and retire. I've been teaching for 25 years and I only have 5 more to go.

Dr. Caso: I don't earn money here. I just participate. I'm a free assistant in Hospital X_____, also without pay. I work there three days a week, Monday mornings, Wednesdays, and Fridays. In the afternoons I'm in my office from five to eight. I'm also the head instructor of psychiatric semiology for third year medicine. I have a title and I earn a little, but just during the school year. I'm also a professor of a hygiene course for the first year of social work, and I teach a course on pathology for the second year. I also have a course on family education in Y_____ University. I have a course on psychology and mental hygiene in the public health nursing program for graduate nurses. It's in the Ministry of Public Health. I'm also a professor in a course on psychiatry for nurses in the nursing school at the Hospital Z_____. In Hospital A_____ I also teach a course for first year nurses. From all that teaching I earn from S/.1,200 to 1,300 a month. I get very little from my office practice, around S/.1,500 a month. It varies but that's all. I don't have any other resources.

Dr. Díaz: I'm assistant physician in my pavilion and they pay me S/.850 a month. Then I'm an assistant in the Department of Psychiatry in Hospital X_____ where I work three hours a day. The salary is S/.5,000. I'm also a professor of the psychology of learning in a university, for which I receive S/.900. I'm a teacher of projective techniques in the same institute and so I get another S/.900. Then I'm an assistant professor of general and experimental psychology in another university. I work in my office three days a week, from five to eight. It's about nine hours. Patients often make an appointment and don't come. I also work in X_____ Clinic where I'm resident physician two days a week. I stay there for twenty-four hours on Saturdays and leave at seven in the evening on Tuesdays. I earn about S/.10-12,000 a month.

Dr. Espinoza: I'm a free participant here, without pay. I come every day from nine to twelve. I'm consulting physician in psychiatry and neurology at Hospital X_____. It's also work with no pay. I come when they call me. I'm also physician for a mutual association of teachers, also in the specialty of psychiatry. I change them per consultation. It comes to S/.70 per patient. I've been teaching a course for the students in the third year of medicine for the last two years. My title is Head of Practice for Psychiatric Semiology. It's two hours a week, in neurology for September and October and in psychiatry for the rest of the year. The pay is very little, an honorarium of S/.566. I don't have any other income, except from my own office; but that's variable. In March, July, and December clients are scarce, except for emergencies. I take care of middle-class people who generally put their money into their children's education. My income is very low, not over S/.12,000.

Dr. Gómez: I'm assistant physician here and I don't earn anything from it. I'm resident physician at the X_____ Clinic. There are four of us and we work by turn, according to when they need us. Today I'm going there to spend the rest of the day, but other days I can only stay for three or four hours. The basic stipend is S/.1,200 with a percentage of the treatments. For example, electroshock costs S/.70 and the resident receives between three and four per cent. Insulin treatment is the same, and S/.1 for every inpatient. We have betwen forty and fifty-five and each one gives us S/.4 or 5. There are also examinations and clinical histories, for which we receive complete fees, S/.200 for an examination and clinical history. Then there are home visits, for which we get S/.650 for picking up a patient; and we get a nurse, a car, and so forth. With all of that I earn between S/.4 and 5,000 in addition to the stipend. It's an open clinic; anyone can bring his patients there. If I bring one, I get thirty per cent in addition to the treatments. If a doctor from the street brings a patient, he also earns his thirty per cent. Then I'm also professor of general psychology in Y_____ University. The pay is S/.200 a month. It's another title and another experience. I go there two hours a week. I also teach a course in sociology here in the School of Nursing. It consists of twenty classes and I earn S/.20 for each one. In total, my income comes to S/.7,000, with 1,000 for consultations, and 2,000 when it's good. I don't have any other occupations.

Dr. Ibarra: I work here in two pavilions as a voluntary participant. Recently in my medical career, I've held the job of professor of biological sciences and psychology in secondary institutions. Currently, I'm a physician doing professional work. I'm also head of practice in neuro-anatomy and clinical head in the psychiatric chair in the Faculty of Medicine in X___ University. I don't have any other occupation.

The physician's economic situation is hardly a secret in Peru, but then neither is the poverty associated with the practice of other professions which demand much less from their practitioners. It is a tribute to these doctors' dedication, devotion, and persistence that they continued to practice their specialty with dignity and enthusiasm. While they did not lose sight of the practical issues of making a living, nor did they eschew aspirations for a rich and meaningful existence for themselves and their families, they also expressed selfless interests in helping people and in scientific research. This is clear in their responses to the question of why they chose their careers:

> Dr. Alba: I discovered my vocation when I was studying medicine. I studied medicine for the purpose of being a psychiatrist; that is, I wanted to be a psychiatrist before I studied medicine. In my third year of high school I took a course in psychology and my interest continued from that time.

> Dr. Bueno: I always liked philosophy. My reason for being a teacher was a great influence for me to understand human structure, physically and mentally. And it was also because there are so many cases of illness where people die without control, in the hands of herbalists or curers. And, above all, they taught us psychological testing in normal school. The instructor demonstrated how those tests were constructed. So the only way for me was to satisfy that desire by entering the Faculty of Medicine. And also that was my mother's desire when I was little.

> Dr. Chávez: In my household I looked at my sisters who were nurses. They worked in medical services, and they told me that a doctor was a high person in cultural matters, a more respected person, more than in other professions. Every time I got sick, I wanted to treat myself. After I got into medicine, I wanted to know the true meaning of people's souls. I wanted to uncover their thinking. I felt strange among other people by my own way of being. I was sad because people who listened to me were not like I was. I was sincere, frank, without malice. I asked why all the others around me were not like that.

> Dr. Díaz: Because I had great interest in the wellbeing of people. I believed that I could do much good, not just for individuals themselves but for humanity. I've been like that since I was very small. I took all the science courses there were in high school and I

got good grades. My worst grades were in deportment. Psychology interested me. When I was in college I did a lot of work in the biological sciences. I can't say exactly why I chose psychology. I've also liked visiting hospitals since I was a child.

Dr. Espinoza: It was my vocation from the time I was a boy. I had two vocations, actually: medicine and engineering. I was teaching primary school and I saw that medicine was more interesting, and socially more important. It's a paradox that I chose the psychological branch. I preferred surgery, but when the student comes to the sixth year there are two courses, neurology and psychiatry. I went to my *paisano* [i.e., person from the same locality], Dr. Fernández, to get some advice. And afterward I stayed with him until now because he was the head there.

Dr. Fernández: I liked it. It was a vocation, a favorite pastime, since I was in high school. I was studying to be a priest, but it didn't attract me. I always admired physicians and their profession, especially the cultural level that one can reach in that environment. That attracted me most. I thought that physicians were doing a lot of good, and that they were reaching an elevated intellectual position. That happened to me after I had left the seminary. There is much relationship between the seminary and my present career of curing souls. In reality, I'm still a lay priest. I viewed the study of medicine as a dream. I never thought I'd arrive because it was a material impossibility. We were poor in those years. My idea was just an idea, nothing more. But when I finished high school, by chance, I wrote to a rich uncle and he offered to help me a little. He give me thirty soles a month. That was enough for a modest life, and with that I got ready to enter the university. I came to Lima to study medicine and also to look for work.

Dr. Gómez: I always liked research. I thought it would be better in medicine. I wanted to study mental and psychological matters. I chose psychiatry and I had to take medicine.

Dr. Herrera: I didn't choose the career of medicine, because choosing means deciding among various possibilities. The career of medicine was the only goal I set for myself since I knew that I had to prepare for some kind of productive activity. Undoubtedly, I must include identification with my father who was an understanding and competent physician.

Dr. Ibarra: Because I liked the biological science from the time I had my secondary education. Because from that time on I thought medicine was the best of all careers, and the most complete. And because an intense feeling for humanity moved me.

Dr. Jara: Those were my father's wishes, which he let me know from the time I was little. Later they became mine.

Dr. López: I chose to study medicine because it was what was more in agreement with my fundamentally scientific interests, expecially chemistry. My motivation wasn't oriented especially by the desire to acquire a therapeutic or a surgical skill in order to earn a living, but, rather, because in medicine there was an exciting field of action for someone who liked the sciences.

Professional training takes place in a larger context than formal higher education, and much of it is personal, informal, and outside the marketplace. Indeed, the doctors depended on these reciprocities to make up for their poverty and the deficiencies in their training; thus, good relations with colleagues had high priority. Here are my notes of a conversation with Dr. Méndez:

Dr. Méndez talked about his training. He came to Larco Herrera with Dr. Alba and others. He worked under Dr. Lleras who not only taught formally but had his students come to his home on Wednesday nights for supper. Sometimes they would stay till two in the morning. Dr. Lleras would read books in English and translate them. He made his library open to the students. Dr. Méndez feels that Dr. Lleras has been a great master.

Dr. Bueno told me:

I am very grateful to Dr. Obregón for the way in which he carries on psychiatry in his pavilion, and because he has continually offered me opportunities to overcome a series of problems. I have received wise advice from him.

Dr. Gómez said:

My entry here was very special. I came without knowing a single physician. I wanted to get to know the place and to work here. I came one afternoon during a vacation to see Dr. Romero who was the

> resident. I told him that I was interested and that I would read. He offered to take me to see the patients. He gave me books to read. Later I came to know other physicians and to to into the pavilions. That was the way I got to know the Hospital.

When I asked the doctors, "Are you satisfied with your preparation for the work you are doing?," not one provided an unqualified positive response. Most indicated with some detail their felt lacks or needs. Here are some of their responses:

> Dr. Alba: Nobody is satisfied. My basic preparation is not enough. I think that one can fill the empty spaces if one is conscious of this limitation and tries to overcome it.

> Dr. Bueno: I began my training in another pavilion. It happened that, with regard to these problems of treatment, I utilized tranquility and reading to overcome on my own a series of problems. It's because books don't get bothered or annoyed, and one always finds a good understanding and a good orientation in any book. Still, I'm not happy with my current preparation. There is much to learn about in other fields of knowledge and experience, in all a series of problems that can be useful to a person. I also feel satisfaction in being able to handle psychiatric matters with the modest psychiatric preparation that I possess. Of course, it is very interesting to travel to other places to learn and orient oneself better in psychiatric science.

> Dr. Caso: I was not trained in a center designed for the formation of specialists. I'm not totally satisfied. For example, I'm lacking training in pathological anatomy related to my specialty. Then there are problems of access to bibliography, like books and journals. Some students look at the phenomenological and others have a more psychoanalytic orientation. I'm here with the first group, but I look at both sides. There's a third group. I'm not in any. I think of myself as eclectic.

> Dr. Díaz: No. In no way. We lack psychological training, and anthropological and sociological orientations. When I was a student there was a lack of cases that we see every day. They gave us many rare and exotic cases from the old asylums. That gives the student the idea that it is strange when in reality it's most human. Then senior people forget to help their juniors, to increase their knowledge. There's much selfishness here.

Dr. Espinoza: My stay here is for getting trained. One can develop oneself in other places, too. Without a doubt, yes, I'm satisfied. One does not come out of it with security, but one acquires the capacity to deal with any problem.

Dr. Fernández: I'm very busy and that interferes with reading. There's too much to do. I like very much to read about different things, but time is hard to find. In this sense, I'm not satisfied with myself. I'd like to have my work and have time to keep on learning. I have to work in order to satisfy my needs. Otherwise, how would I live? To read and write, I'd have to stay up all night. I use Sundays and holidays for doing scientific work. I work with legal cases, making decisions for judges. Sometimes I receive a small stipend for this, if the government has funds. Most of the time it's without pay and it takes a lot of time.

Dr. Gómez: Preparation in itself won't give me professional qualifications. My colleagues will give it to me. Dr. Pérez, Dr. Lleras and Dr. Quesada were practically my professors. When I got to the course on psychiatry, I already knew it. They had already been supervising my practice and my reading for two or three years. Courses are very limited and one doesn't learn very much.

Dr. Ibarra: No. A sensation of imperfection is evident to me. I'd like to have further training in foreign countries.

Dr. Jara: For the time being, yes, but for future work I'm thinking about including even more training.

Dr. López: In no way. I think that my basic preparation and my psychiatric knowledge leave much to be desired. Most especially, I am sorry not to have greater knowledge in neurophysiology, biochemistry, psychoanalysis, and psychotherapy in general.

Despite the lacks they felt in their training, the doctors clearly articulated high standards of psychiatric practice. They expected psychiatrists to have a thorough grounding in the science of medicine without neglecting their spiritual development. They wished members of their profession, thus, to be humanists but also to possess a persistent scientific curiosity about human conditions. Moreover, they expected their colleagues to exert control over their own selves and be open to other persons. While this reflects expectations absorbed during their training and, so, of course, a degree of professionalization, the twelve professionals all responded as individuals to my question of what qualifications one should have to be a psychiatrist:

> Dr. Alba: First, a rather balanced motivation, a quite constant emotional life. One ought to be a person with few affective problems. Second, an acute capacity for observation in order to evaluate clinical facts adequately. I think that this is the most important capacity. Third, an acceptable biological and medical culture, and a certain literary, social, and philosophical culture. Fourth, a capacity for understanding the alien soul, and for participating in the troubles and problems of others.
>
> Dr. Bueno: Broad culture from the humanistic point of view. Then, a wide general medical knowledge. One must know sociology, psychology, and, of course, psychopathology; and one must have aptitudes for those. And one must be a constant and persevering person, responsible for one's actions, one who tries to be a model, that is, to serve as an example for others.
>
> Dr. Caso: To be a psychiatrist, as in all specialties, one needs to have at least an average intelligence. It's important to have unbiased and balanced judgment. Then to be an observer but not only of the most obvious things. Also, one should not be just a practicing physician but one should devote oneself to study. The psychiatrist has to study more than in other specialties.
>
> Dr. Chávez: There are two basic skills: one should more or less understand oneself; and at the same time one should understand the other person during a clinical interview. That is basic for me. One should have moral and spiritual support in order to comprehend the person adequately in all aspects. I don't like hypocrisy.
>
> Dr. Díaz: One should receive adequate training, which one doesn't get in the Faculty of Medicine. Everybody gets it according to their tendencies and needs. It should be an idea of the group that is not just theoretical. Everybody goes off alone.
>
> Dr. Espinoza: The psychiatrist has to be a general clinician. One ought to know the clinical part well, and to understand the neurological bases. One should have a humanistic culture. Then one can begin in the field of psychiatry. Then one can approach the psychophysical reality of the patient.

Dr Fernández: The psychiatrist ought to have an honest character, morality in all things, a spirit of understanding, patience, tolerance, cordiality, human feeling, knowledge of his own spirit, general culture, and a spirit of sacrifice.

Dr. Gómez: In the first place, a medical vocation. In the second place, one ought to have culture in the wide sense of the word. In the third place, a rather balanced personality.

Dr. Herrera: Above average intelligence. Sufficient theoretical and technical training. Persistence for continuing to improve and widening one's knowledge over the whole course of one's life. A sincere desire to do humanitarian and educational work, but not necessarily in teaching. A set of values defined and oriented toward worthy objects. Beyond these requirements, I think that a psychiatrist should combine the following: the ability to communicate on all levels, psychological sensitivity and delicacy, and a personality that is free from those disturbances that could prevent the effective exercise of psychotherapy.

Dr. Ibarra: A great feeling for humanity, a solid scientific preparation, high intelligence, responsibility, and morality, a capacity for serene judgment, an interest in scientific research, humanistic culture, understanding of the human soul, and the capacity for intuiting the psyche.

Dr. Jara: The gift of sympathy with human beings, especially with patients. A wide discernment for understanding human problems and exploring them in depth as a totality. And as great an inclination for the natural sciences as for the spiritual sciences.

Dr. López: Being sufficiently prepared in the basic sciences, having enough experience in medicine and surgery, having a prolonged and varied training with psychiatric patients, posessing certain personal characteristics like intelligence, good judgment, sensitivity and respect for the alien soul, and interest in people and their social and family life, and, finally, a desire to study and improve oneself continually.

The individuality of these doctors showed up even more strongly when they were asked to state their preferences in regard to professional tasks and the kinds of patients they saw; but there also appeared in the interviews a patterned need for work in which the positive results of their labors could be observed, which could be less an indication of personal weakness and more an indication of the state of their profession:

> Dr. Alba: I like scientific research the most. Among my duties, I like the clinical study of patients. What I like least are the administrative aspects. We lose much time that way which could be used to help patients. I am more interested in psychosis, especially in schizophrenia. I want to do research on that. I also like to work with a patient who is more capable to describe what he feels, one with a deeper knowledge who can offer a picture of his abnormal experiences. I have less interest in the very deeply mentally retarded, those who have serious intellectual defects.

> Dr. Bueno: I have more interest in treatment and in psychological testing, because the patient's improvement depends on treatment and, of course, together with clinical practice which is the mother of medicine. Without knowing the patient one could not do anything. But I have to see everything. If there were other physicians who could take charge of the other things, I would devote myself to the clinic, to treatment, and to testing. Research charms me a lot. I don't like the administrative aspects. Why study medicine for that? Students of economics can take charge of that. I prefer child patients, probably because of my training in education. And middle-aged patients, because it's necessary to keep up their health as a factor that helps in many aspects of family life. Then older patients because we are all of us going there. One grows old and nobody cares if they treat one badly. One has to be very human with old age and with youth. I have less interest in the mentally retarded, because they are not capable of communicating what they feel, and the deepest ones constitute a social burden. It would be better to practice euthanasia in this case.

> Dr. Caso: There is just one aspect I like most, and that is to observe one patient all morning. Sometimes I'm required to see all of them. Then I like teaching more than practice. Practice can be done as an instrument for teaching, and that is because I have taken on too many hours, even though it's an economic disadvantage. I prefer neurotic patients because it's something more like normal, closer, where the environment is very influential. It's more understandable. I have less interest in the rest, but that doesn't mean that our attention to them repels me.

Dr. Chávez: I like the clinical part, nosology. I need to see those things. With regard to patients, I've always asked myself which I prefer. All people who need medical service should be helped in breadth by the physician, and without reservations. Among mental patients, they all interest me, because for me the task is that the physician should always extend himself to patients. One has to try to help, when there is one who is disturbed, to reduce symptoms, have him understand with the means that exist. I don't know why I'm always affectionate. I try to get close to them. I try to be careful not to hurt them. I have a patient whom I'm trying to raise. He has almost no defenses. I want to put him in contact with reality, make jokes with him, play with him. He's improving.

Dr. Díaz: My tasks are varied and I have wide liberty. I have no preference, as long as things are doing like that. My ideal work would be research and teaching. I prefer the intelligent neurotic patient, not the psychotic, because I see that I am useless in the Hospital. There are so many things that it lacks.

Dr. Espinoza: I prefer outpatients, the new patients on Mondays and Saturdays, because there one acquires more diagnostic capability and more experience in treatment. I like patients who present neurosis because they are easier patients, self-observers in whom psychological phenomena can be seen in depth. I like the cerebral organic patients least. They're less productive.

Dr. Fernández: I have more interest in the attention and treatment of patients and the preparation of cases for teaching. We are experimenting with new drugs from outside that the pharmaceutical companies send us. I especially like acute cases because they are the ones which can benefit the most from what we have to offer. I have less interest in patients who are very disorganized mentally, in the very advanced mentally retarded.

Dr. Gómez: For me the ideal would be research and, in the second place, teaching. I don't like private consultation very much. I prefer the acute type of patients because in them there are possibilities for treatment and recuperation. I like the irrecuperable less, especially the mentally retarded. I've asked myself why I don't like them. They can be productive in occupational therapy, and then, perhaps, we might like them. Right now they are worthless because of the lack of means.

Dr. Herrera: I have no preference for any aspect of the tasks I carry out because all of them, more or less effectively, tend toward the desired objective. I don't have any preference in regard to the kind of patient, but it's more pleasant to work with acute cases. I'd rather attend psychotics in the Hospital and neurotics in my private practice. I have less interest in those for whom my labors have less chance of being effective.

Dr. Ibarra: Professional practice in the hospital environment. Psychological research and experimentation, psychopathology. University teaching. Reading in general. And in my free time, the practice of drawing and painting.

Dr. Jara: Research in psychopathology and psychotherapy, especially in psychosis and research on body constitution.

Dr. López: Teaching and research. I would prefer to work in a general university hospital where I could develop intensive work in study and teaching within a comprehensive plan of interchange with the other departments of the hospital. I'd also like to work in editorial and literary activities. I prefer the intelligent and differentiated patient who is capable of permitting a good exploration and following orders comfortably. I have less interest in patients with language disturbances, the mentally retarded, and certain types of neurotics.

I asked the doctors to define a "mental hospital" and to define the purpose of the Hospital Víctor Larco Herrera. In their responses the distinction between the ideals absorbed in the course of their professional training and real conditions is easily to be observed:

Dr. Alba: The mental hospital is the specialized part of medicine which has for its object the study and treatment of behavioral disorders in their most varied expressions. And basic research on mental disorders. All the pavilions have the same goal, the study of the patient and his treatment; but these are different. A pavilion for the chronic type has a custodial service. In others more is done in regard to the study and active treatment in order to try to reintegrate the patient into the community with the best functioning of his personality.

Dr. Bueno: A mental hospital is a place for the recuperation of patients who are suffering from a mental illness. This Hospital should

have all the pavilions working to develop a rivalry among the different ones in order to elevate to the maximum the progress of psychiatry in the national scene.

Dr. Caso: The mental hospital is a hospital that is distinguished because patients with mental disturbances are treated in it. In a general sense, this Hospital should care for patients as much as possible, both internal patients and outpatients. There exist limitations in this attention, for example, economic ones because sometimes there are not enough medications. Then personnel is another problem. Currently, this one is the only mental hospital in the country. We are not proud of this, because there ought to be others.

Dr. Chávez: A mental hospital is an institution where various mental disturbances are treated, primarily in relation to the upsets which these patients cause in society or in their households. We see that this is a hospital something like a kind of asylum. I don't know: for me it ought to have a medical staff that should concern itself that the patients get out of here quickly, and also that, in the same way, those outside can find space in here. There should be movement.

Dr. Díaz: A mental hospital is a center of which there are two types, one that is active for acute patients, and another for chronic patients. The first should be a center for reintegration, with a prophylactic function, and the second should be a more moderate place where patients can live. Many people would come looking for help with confidence. Here in Peru people try to hide it. This Hospital ought to disappear. The whole system ought to disappear. There shouldn't even be a reorganization. It should be done from the beginning.

Dr. Espinoza: At least in our medium, a mental hospital is the place where attention is given both to acute and chronic patients, among persons with mental illnesses. Simply the fact that it is a special service means that this Hospital has to provide everything that is needed for the best treatment of psychiatric patients. In this sense it should begin by having good personnel. Then it should take up patient care and research labors with the greatest economy.

Dr. Fernández: Here in Peru the Hospital is the place where care is given to patients who present serious alterations in behavior. This Hospital, according to those who built it, should serve as depository for chronic patients. But this is neither desirable nor what current circumstances require. There are many mental patients, including acute ones, who ought to be interned for their own benefit, which is accomplished only with great difficulty because of the orientation which Hospital authorities have. This places great limits on the benefits that can be achieved, unless we had the liberty to admit or hospitalize those acute patients who urgently need isolation from family environment and treatment. Currently, we are reluctantly complying with the orientation imposed on us and we do not look very sympathetically on the admission of patients on the basis of personal connections.

Dr. Gómez: The mental hospital is a specialized place for the care and treatment of illnesses of that type. I'm not in agreement with the concept of a psychiatric hospital but with units that give assistance. The real function of the mental hospital is treatment. And there ought to be another kind, the asylum, for chronic cases where they can work. Mental hospitals don't have to be big places. There should be treatment units that could be distributed among the administrative units of the city. The Hospital Victor Larco Herrera is different, currently, from the kind that one might desire. There is great discrimination between patients who pay and those who do not. Ninety-five per cent of those who pay can be of any type, chronic, acute, mentally retarded, psychomanic. They are the great majority who stay in the Hospital. On the other hand, we are limited in admitting people who really need treatment, possible short-term, which could produce recuperation. There was a case of a boy of nineteen in catatonic agitation. He came one Saturday and I saw that his condition would need three or four months. I signed the papers but they would not let him in. The next week he burned down his mother's house.

Dr. Herrera: A mental hospital is a corporate association of physicians, technical personnel. administrative personnel, and auxilliary personnel who, supplied with sufficient technical means, serve in order to give individualized and specialized attention to a more or less fixed number of internal or ambulatory patients who suffer from mental disturbances in a broad sense. The fundamental objectives of the hospital have to be directed at the etiological treatment of illness, the provision of attention to internal patients who are currently incurable, and being the center of a social and individual educative labor. The mental hospital may or may not be related to instruction, but it is suitable that such a relationship exist and that it be a close one. The same thing can be said about research. The

Hospital Victor Larco Herrera should give attention to the maximum number of patients possible, both internal and outpatients. After a total reorganization, that would include the replacement of certain departments and pavilions by others that were appropriately equipped, and that would take into account the economic reality of all those who worked or attended in it, the Hospital should be converted into a center of attention and instruction of much greater breadth and based more in accord with current psychiatric criteria.

Dr. Ibarra: A mental hospital is an establishment devoted to the treatment of insane patients and which, for such purposes, studies with multidimensional criteria the sick person, and then carries out the most adequate therapy and tries to place him in an optimum state of mental health or make possible his life with others in society. In our Hospital patients from almost all over the country are treated, because it is the only specialized one. It should be able to count on greater material resources for the benefit of the great number of patients it shelters.

Dr. Jara: The mental hospital is a community of patients, physicians, and auxilliary personnel, in which there is the effort to give the first, by means of adequate somatic and psychotherapeutic treatment, a style of life comparable to that which normal people enjoy who live in normal communities. This Hospital achieves in a very limited way some part of the care and treatment of mental patients in the several pavilions with internal patients and in outpatient consultation with ambulatory ones.

Dr. López: A mental hospital is an institution designed for the rehabilitation of the mental patient in all aspects, somatic, psychic, and social. Its function of custody and asylum should be passed on to other organizations. This Hospital ought to achieve a labor of national scope, taking into account that it is the only psychiatric hospital in the country. It should accomplish its labor of treatment, research, and instruction, through the solidary action of all its physicians, something that is not happening.

Finally, I asked the panel of respondents, "If I were a medical student or a new doctor here, what advice would you give me to get along?" They answered:

Dr. Alba: First, I'd advise you to live a little of the daily experience of the patient so that you'd get used to thinking that the mental patient is different from us in only a few aspects. We have to experience the twenty-four hours of the patient. Second, to examine with the greatest ingenuity and simplicity the patients' disturbances and then discuss this reality in relation to the content of texts, so as to be able to judge the books in terms of the patient's reality. I'd tell you this with more emphasis because we all have the tendency to see reality through books instead of the reverse. Third and last, to have patience, much patience, to deal with your patients, to study them, understand them, and to be a psychiatrist, because psychiatry is a road that one has to travel without hurry.

Dr. Bueno: To relate to patients frequently, observe each one of them, because each patient is a small world which needs to be known from very close. Then to be consistent and persevering in relations between the physician and the patient. And, of course, to come to the pavilion, to the Hospital. Another aspect would be reading, the management of general psychology, medical and psychological pathology, sociology, because these are the areas which help one in one's professional formation. Another thing would be to tell you to look for the psychiatrist with whom you can place a certain affinity in personal communication and for the degree of your preparation.

Dr. Caso: Really, I would tell you in detail about the parts of the pavilion, the organization, both the material and the psychological aspects, the patients and the personnel who attend them. I'm not the kind of friend to give something else. This would be the best service to you, to inform you on everything possible. I'm not interested in giving a list of advice.

Dr. Chávez: More than anything else, balance in your emotional state, constant reading daily, good will, perseverence, consistency and discipline in work. And to take, if it is possible, twelve hours at work.

Dr. Díaz: [He laughs.] I was going to say that, if you were from some other country, you should go home as soon as possible. Seriously, I'd give you specific information, teach you everything that happened to me. Many new people are up in the air and find it disorienting. They don't know how to do things. I'd teach you the fundamentals.

Dr. Espinoza: When one arrives, its the way to make contact with a patient. During the first days, one should have an expectant attitude. Later, through one's own initiative, one can approach a patient taking all necessary precautions. Second, I'd let you know the way in which activities take place in the pavilion in order to avoid any conflict with the other medical personnel. Third, I'd suggest punctuality and interest in the patients who are in your care.

Dr. Fernández: If you are a specialist, you already know how to care for patients. I'd tell you about the kinds of patients here with their respective personalities, the patients' customs, the kind of personnel we have, and the peculiarities of the physicians who are already working in the hospital, so as to favor everybody's adjustment. I'd tell you the same about the patients, and the days and hours for treatments.

Dr. Gómez: In the first place, to spend as much time as possible in the Hospital. Second, to see the patients candidly without any prejudice, either what is common among the majority of people or what the books have to say. Third, to dedicate yourself to a specific patient, to study him as well as you can, in detail, and then to go from the patient to books and then from books to the patient. And to try to maintain the greatest harmony with all of your colleagues and to work within the Hospital's discipline.

Dr. Herrera: The advice that can be given to a person so he can adapt to a specific state of things depends fundamentally on his mode of being, his goals, his preparation, and so forth. Since I don't know you, it's impossible for me to give you any advice.

Dr. Ibarra: That you ignore the material and even technical deficiencies which exist in our Hospital. That, apart from your clinical tasks, you investigate and learn about our social and cultural medium.

Dr. Jara: The cultivation of prudence, patience, compassion, the gift of humanity, and depth in observation.

Dr. López: To study most profoundly, to maintain a lively interest in patients as persons and fellow humans, and to maintain close personal and scientific relations with the other physicians in the Hospital.

Despite the grim realities of psychiatric practice in Peru, the poverty and the constriction this poverty imposes on one who endeavors to alleviate pain, suffering, and misery, the images which emerge from these professional responses show great optimism. From them I am drawn to the conclusion that despite the great odds against the successful outcome of their interventions, the doctors refused to stop trying to heal. They showed lively interest in knowing their patients as human beings, desire for breadth and depth of knowledge, willingness to know and live with themselves, and enthusiasm in their exchanges with their colleagues. In no way were they defeated by the desperate environment in which they lived. Because they shared the myth that "things get better," and because they insisted on correcting reality instead of merely understanding it, they seemed to be, more than optimists, true revolutionaries. José Carlos Mariátegui (1959:28) could as easily have said of them, as he said of revolutionary spirits: "The attitude of the man who proposes to correct reality is, certainly, more optimistic than pessimistic. He is a pessimist in his protest and in his condemnation of the present; but he is an optimist in his hope for the future." The spirit of Peruvian psychiatry is articulated well by Javier Mariátegui Chiappe (1988:23) who confronts his national realities by rejecting "its passive examination and, even more, its resigned conformism." Rather, he adds, "we should move toward its correction, imbued with optimistic voluntarism to rectify errors of the past." In this we see the images of the healers of the 1959 research who were guided by their myth. However, they were neither dreamers nor tricksters--although, to be sure, it is clear that they had not given up the pursuit of their dreams, nor had they yielded up their vision of the magical power of the human spirit--but scientists committed to researching the workings of the material and spiritual universe of humanity in order to make that universe a better place for themselves and their fellow human beings.

Notes

1. In Peru, a public charity society (*beneficencia pública*) is an association of prominent persons which supervises a number of charitable enterprises like hospitals, orphanages, special schools, and other benevolent institutions. It is subsidized partly by public funds and partly by private donations.

2. A Bolivian psychiatrist, Mario Argandoña (*in* Alarcón 1990:97-98) describes the economic problems of practice in his country in a statement which could just as easily apply in Peru: "They have just approved a budget in Bolivia which increases excessively, for me and for the greatest part of public

opinion, the budget for the armed forces. It turns out that now a Bolivian with the rank of army colonel earns more than a thousand dollars. In contrast, the Rector of the University makes two hundred dollars, and a physician in the Ministry makes 50 to 70 dollars. This very much discourages institutional and social practice, because social practice can't be performed with compensation, the government has to pay your social security, and the salary of the paramedical worker has to come from the State. So what is the result of having a miserable salary? Private practice, and you give it a lot of attention, you do it with real dedication and effort because you live on it. In Cochabamba, with daily office hours, you get 5 dollars, and with a month of that 150 dollars. So you're making what a rector gets. If you have a hospitalized patient, you can easily reach 500 dollars. Well, here is a real problematic, which is that the State doesn't support social practice. Social practice means . . . taking care of poor people who can't pay; but somebody has to pay for it because the physician, after his studies, his preparation, has relatively high expectations. The physician, the psychiatrist, is not going to live exactly like the traditional Andean psychiatrist, the *aysiri* and the *jampiri* [folk practioners] who really live quite frugally. The physician has certain needs for consumption that you're not going to take away from him, either. So undoubtedly private practice in Bolivia is the principal source of support for physicians, and this private practice undoubtedly favors the classes that can pay for it. . . . In the psychiatric hospital, San Juan de Dios, in the last few months, each patient has lost on the average 12 kilos of weight; and the physicians have to be permanently on strike because they are in almost the same condition as the patients, on the verge of starving to death."

3. "Poor" is a good adjective to use in describing physicians, especially those who are in the process of establishing themselves. The mature psychiatrists in my sample, in contrast, belong to a Peruvian income-earning elite, according to Webb (1977:13), since an annual income of the equivalent of $5,000 places them in the top 1%, "a group of about 30,000 people with incomes above $2,600."

Chapter 2

Concepts of Mental Illness Held by the Hospital Population.

This chapter deals with one part of a series of informal question schedules with which I interviewed the different population categories of the Hospital Víctor Larco Herrera. The schedule dealt with the varied perspectives of these people regarding hospital life, values, goals, and beliefs. Although psychiatric facilities in Peru have changed much during the more than thirty years which intervened between the original research and this report (see Mariátegui Chiappe 1988), it is possible that the data can still communicate something new to colleagues who are interested in the structures and processes of psychiatric facilities, and how to make them more effective; and so it is worth the effort to analyze them. This Chapter is based on a question about the concepts of mental illness expressed by the psychiatrists, clinical psychologists, social workers, nurses, aides, and patients who worked or lived in the Hospital. It endeavors to describe this hospital ideology--or, rather, these ideologies--and ventures to draw some conclusions with respect to the way the Hospital functions. The question was: in the case of the psychiatrists, "Please define mental illness briefly"; and in the case of all the other population categories, "What is mental illness? How does it happen? From what does it come?" Only patients in Pavilion 20 were interviewed, but the schedules for the professional and paraprofessional personnel were administered in both Pavilion 20 and other pavilions. There were no differences to be discerned among the responses of the sub-populations of the different pavilions, as we might expect, but there were significant differences among the responses of the different professional, paraprofessional, and patient categories. These relate to social class, ethnic, and educational variables.

I began the research with the goal of studying a mental hospital as one would study any other institutional context; that is, that it was composed of categories of persons, all of whose behaviors and verbalizations had the same weight for anthropological purposes. To a certain degree, this point of view was correct, but for the purposes of writing this Chapter about concepts of mental illness, it was not so. In the first place, I found that, among the patients, the character of the disorder that had brought them into the Hospital had its effects on their responses to the question. There were significant differences between the statements of the schizophrenics who, with the exception of those who had achieved some improvement and had at least a minimum of self-knowledge, demonstrated one or another degree of disorientation, and the rest, including the over- or underproduction of those diagnosed under the category of cyclic emotional disturbances. Thus, while it is possible to include their responses it is also necessary to examine these with clinical reservations.

I also found that the general structure of Peruvian society and culture conditioned the responses. A division clearly showed between the professional persons and the non-professionals. The former, according to their training experiences, shared ideas to the point where the popular ideology of mental health and illness does not appear. This is especially noteworthy among the nurses whose origins are located in the popular strata. In contrast, the attendants who were all of Andean origin responded almost totally in popular terms. The patients, too, tended to respond in popular terms, although their therapeutic experiences are to be seen in many of their other statements (see Chapter 4). It seems to me that this illustrates very well the unconscious exclusion[1] of popular strata from the ideas of middle strata, reflected in the training (or lack of it) of attendants, of whom the expectation did not exist that they would have some role to play in the construction of therapy. Consequently, it is necessary to examine the medical concepts of Andean popular culture in order to compare paraprofessionals with professionals.

Custred (1979:297) notes the difference between the vision of the spiritual and the material of European-Christian tradition and Andean tradition:

> The soul of a person is his essence, that is the constellation of attributes which account for the life and the character of individual human beings. Different cultural traditions weigh the behavioral, the emotional, the intellectual and the physical attributes of Man in different ways in the formation of their divergent soul concepts, thus revealing to the ethnologist a wide range of variation. These variations in turn appear to be based on two broad conceptual themes. One is seen in the Christian doctrine where the spiritual and the material are conceptionally opposed to one another to form two distinct spheres of reality, with the spiritual always presiding over the material, where matter and spirit are two rarely separable aspects of the same thing. . . . Since matter and spirit are dichotomous realities in the Christian tradition, the Latin and the Spanish terms for "body" and "soul" stand in a semantic relationship of opposition to one another, thus reflecting in lexical usage the conceptual opposition which underlies it. . . . In pre-hispanic Quechua, however, such a semantic relationship could not have existed since the central concept of soul was thought to be the potencies of corporeal organs, not some totally opposed spiritual force, and since the free soul seems to have been of a dual nature, each soul expressing perhaps two distinct sets of human or individual personality characteristics which were split up after death. Furthermore, there is evidence to suggest that there did not even exist a single word for body in the Spanish sense of the term.

In the nearly five hundred years since the Spanish conquest of Peru, there have been deep changes in Andean ideology; but it should be pointed out that contemporary Andean culture is syncretistic, originating in two traditions. In Andean folk beliefs, the ideology of the inseparability of body and spirit is still to be discerned; and from the point of view of an Andean curer the causes of an illness appear in the total life of a patient, rather than in the presentation of a clinical case. Chiappe Costa (1979:80) indicates that "for curers, the characteristics of the illness are defined more by its etiology than by its clinical or symptomatological manifestations." According to Chiappe Costa, Lemlij, and Millones (1985:11), that explanation is what is important and what can also have its therapeutic effects: "The patient may or may not get cured, but after the session he will understand the reason for his sickness, thereby reducing the level of his uneasiness." Seguín (1979:39), who has studied the practice of popular medicine intensively and deeply, discusses two major categories of illness, "illnesses from God" and "illnesses from injury," the former of which "are 'natural' illnesses, produced by non-magical factors, understandable as the influence of the forces of nature," while the latter "always have a supernatural origin"; and he adds:

> In the cases we have studied, "injury" appeared in different forms and was attributed to different influences. It is a magical form of action on health and its treatment is also fundamentally magical. If injury is produced by people--because of "envy" and other factors--it acts through a "*Malero*," a malicious witch, and should be cured by liberating the patient from the effects produced by his influence. Thus, the injury can be made "through the mouth," when the subject has been made to ingest some substance which produces in him the alleged ill-omened results, or "through the air," when it is supposed that it has been caused by inhalation. We believe that a special form of "injury" is "soul theft." In this case the pathological influence is not determined by persons but by the elements of nature: a mountain, a river, etc.

Popular medical ideology explains illness with a very wide range of concepts and, in view of the results of this Hospital study, it may be useful to summarize the explanations which the inhabitants of a Lima slum, Andean migrants, offered when they were asked about the origin of illnesses in general by Rotondo (1960:7): bad food, carelessness, contagion, cold, failure to keep clean, a bad life, body disorders, bad cleansing of the mouth and stomach, fatigue, fate, too little sleep, and because God wishes it. Rotondo (ibid.:2) says of the responses which had to do with food, the majority of all responses:

> Our attention was called to the frequent belief that a (supposed) accumulation of non-digested food may be the cause of all kinds of indispositions, that is, what is called "*empacho*" [i.e., "dirty stomach"]. But in addition we noted another very common explanation of illness: that of attributing it to weakness occasioned by a reduced ingestion of food. They think that "bad food" [or "bad feeding"] is a cause of many illnesses from tuberculosis even to mental illnesses.

Professional readers will understand quite well the technical considerations which conditioned the responses of the professional informants, but the responses of the aides, and of some of the patients, should be interpreted in the context of Peruvian popular medicine. To illustrate the popular point of view, I include the account of one patient, Don Pedro Armas[2], who presented himself to me spontaneously in the context of a casual conversation on September 11, 1959. Don Pedro, diagnosed as manic-depressive, was born in the highland city of C___, and migrated to the coastal city of Ch___ as a young man for the purpose of engaging in commercial work. Here is what he told me:

> I got sick in Ch__ when I was an employee of a commercial house there. They treated me for three weeks. Several doctor friends took care of me, but they couldn't make me well. I couldn't sleep. My mind was uncontrolled. I remembered sports when I was young, and I wanted to be in a marathon. I wanted to sing. I didn't want to talk to anybody. A woman friend of mine saw that the doctors weren't doing me any good. She advised my relatives to consult a curer. I was treated for three nights with that form of treatment. I think the medicinal herbs were important. On the third night, I woke up as though out of a dream. I felt well. My doctor friends saw this, that I was well, and after they watched me for two weeks they agreed that I was ready to go back to work again. The treatment that made me well lasted eight years. And then the same symptoms came back again. My family in C___ wondered where to send me. They decided that the best psychiatrists in Peru were in the Hospital Víctor Larco Herrera. The authorities at home agreed and sent me here. That was in 1940. I've been here now for nineteen years and I get short treatments. I've gone out three times, thinking I was well, but the thing repeated itself. In view of all this, I think there are two reasons for my sickness: a *brebaje* [i.e., a "potion'] was given to me to make me sick; or it could also be from too much sex. Meanwhile, I'm still alive. I'm 69 years old.

The psychiatrists

It may be anticipated that the responses of the twelve professional physicians in my sample who specialized in psychiatry answered my question in the context of their medical and psychiatric training and experience, matters of their studies, their relations with their mentors, and, of course, their clinical practice. That was so, but it was evident that this context was anything but uniform. They can be divided at least into three broad groupings: those who place emphasis in their definitions of mental illness on behavior or social behavior; those who emphasize organic factors; and those who prefer to speak in terms of psychological functions. In this, the Lima psychiatrists appear to conform to trends among their colleagues elsewhere, as is quite apparent when they are compared with the three ideological groupings Strauss, et al. (1964:54-57) find among North American psychiatrists: sociotherapists, somatotherapists, and psychotherapists. We will examine the Lima responses in this order.

Three psychiatrists gave me definitions of mental illness relating to behavior or social behavior:

> Dr. Alba: It is an alteration of behavior which makes it difficult or impossible for the person to control himself and to adjust to the social environment.

> Dr. Fernández: It is a disorder of the natural development of behavior, and of the acts of the individual, which incapacitates him or diminishes his capacity in his ordinary relations with the environment.

> Dr. Herrera: Mental illness can be defined as a break or failure in social adjustment. It is indicated by psychological symptoms whose polymorphic etiology has to be sought in the psychophysical totality of the being who is suffering.

Two psychiatrists offered me more or less organic concepts:

> Dr. Bueno: It is a disturbance possibly of the neurons of the encephalic mass which brings forth different pictures in patients, involving both the spirit and the body.

> Dr. Gómez: It is primarily a psychological disturbance with a biochemical or biological base.

The other seven defined mental illness in terms of psychological functions:

> Dr. Caso: Mental illness is a loss of health, or a disequilibrium in the functions of a human being, in which what predominates is the psychological, either in the symptoms or possibly in the etiopathogenesis of the disturbance.

Dr. Chávez: Mental illness is a disorganization of the different human psychic spheres with social, familial, and individual repercusions.

Dr. Díaz: It is a serious psychological derangement in a predisposed subject, induced by certain pressures.

Dr. Espinoza: A disorganization penetrates the core of the personality. This is the shortest general definition.

Dr. Ibarra: In a broad sense mental illness can be considered to be a pathological state which engages, with greater or lesser seriousness, the psychic life of a subject, altering his ego and personality, with organic manifestations more or less evident according to the cases.

Dr. Jara: It's a matter of a disequilibrium of the real person in his totality which brings with it manifestations of physico-chemical, biological, and spiritual alterations, and which is broken loose through physico-chemical and biological disturbances in some cases or by disturbances of the soul or spirit in others.

Dr. Lleras: It consists of very different disturbances which involve the functions of the specific personality. Generally, it consists of agitation and subjective suffering, and greater or lesser disorders in interpersonal relations. Its cause it generally multiple and its study demands a multidimensional attack.

The Clinical Psychologists

Only two psychologists were interviewed, a woman and a man, a very small sample, admittedly, but one which can serve to indicate both some common bases as well as some significant differences in the contexts of the different trainings and practices of the several types of professionals:

Psychologist Aguirre: It's something that attacks man's spiritual part, disadjusting him from the environment in which he lives.

Psychologist Bardales: There is a series of causes. Psychosis in itself is apart from reality. There are delusions, false perceptions. Mental illness would be separate from reality. Nobody knows why. There are some biological causes and some psychological causes.

The Social Workers

Two social workers reponded to the question schedule:

> Social Worker Aparicio: It's a disequilibrium in interpersonal relations, in one's way of life, in one's mode of thinking.

> Social Worker Bermejo: It isn't only a physical sickness but it's one that involves a subject's personality. There are problems with the environment, the family, and with each one of the life situations in which the patient finds himself.

The Nurses

Thirteen nurses were interviewed, six women and seven men, of whom six worked in Pavilion 20. When the interviewing began, it was thought that the social origin of the informant--city or small town, coastal or highland region--might reveal significant differences in the ideology of mental illness, but this was not the case. Although the sample included one nurse from Lima, five from other coastal cities, one from a coastal town, three from highland cities, and three from highland towns, no significant differences in the responses are to be found. Rather, except for one case, that of Nurse Delgado who was born in a coastal town, whose statement in part appears to contain a strain of popular medicine, the responses reflect the training of psychiatric nurses (which all of them had obtained in the School of Nursing located on the grounds of the Hospital Víctor Larco Herrera, in those days the only school of nursing in Peru which specialized in psychiatric nursing) and, possibly, as well, a certain reserve in answering the question. Nevertheless, it is possible to categorize the responses in terms of those nurses who placed emphasis on loss of control, those who defined mental illness psychologically, two nurses, including Nurse Delgado also, who emphasized organic causes, and one more case, that of Nurse Jara, who offered a commentary more than a definition of the concept.

Three nurses give definitions of mental illness as the loss of control which, in view of nurses' concern with maintaining order in their services (see Chapter 7), can be read in such a way as to suggest their self-conceptions as providers of control. For them control was part of the package of nursing care:

Nurse Arruga: They are patients who are not responsible for their acts. A mental patient is a being who loses control of his will, of his acts.

Nurse Bustos: Mental illness is the loss of control of one's will, nothing more.

Nurse Frías: It's disturbance. It's a sick soul where one loses all one's controls. The patient becomes unconscious of his acts.

The majority, seven nurses, dealt with aspects that were more specifically psychological:

Nurse Cruz: It's an abnormality of a person's psyche with different manifestations in one's mode of being, thinking, and existing. That's what I think.

Nurse Chivas: As far as I'm concerned, it's that a person has lost all his reason. It can be temporary or permanent, that is, chronic, as we say.

Nurse Esquivel: It's a disturbance that man suffers in his mind, according to circumstances and motives.

Nurse Godoy: It's the total disequilibrium of the patient. They become disoriented in time and space. In some cases, it's the total loss of memory. Each one lives in his interior world. It's a sickness of the mind.

Nurse Hurtado: It's the psychic disorder of a person.

Nurse Llosa: It's a disturbance of the mind.

Two nurses focused their responses, more or less, on organic factors:

Nurse Delgado: It's a disequilibrium of the nervous system, because of which a subject reacts in different ways. In some cases one has light psychomotor excitement and in others it's deep. Disequilibrium comes from some family misadventure, an argument, syphilis, tuberculosis, or from deficient food or traumatisms.

Nurse Lozada: It's a disturbance of the mind produced by different causes. There are disturbances that are hereditary, or metabolic, or that come from intoxications, and so forth.

And, finally, there was one response that defies classification:

> Nurse Justo: It's a very sad sickness.

The Attendants

The interviewing included seventeen attendants, thirteen of them in Pavilion 20 and five in other pavilions, thirteen men and four women. At the beginning, also, it was thought that factors of urbanism, ruralism, and ethnicity might produce conceptual differences, but it turned out that everyone in this group was originally Andean, not creole, for they all originated in small towns and hamlets in the highlands: six from the Department of Cajamarca, three from Amazonas, two from La Libertad, two from Lima [i.e., the Department, not the city], one from Ancash, one from Apurímac, one from Huánuco, and one from San Martín. It is apparent that the "ruling ideology" [i.e., psychiatric understandings] of mental health and illness enters into the responses, undoubtedly leaking in from the Hospital environment, but we easily discern many popular ideas in them. Eleven attendants defined mental illness in terms of a disturbance of the head, of thoughts, or of ideas. Four viewed it as the loss of one or another psychic function. And one said that it was ordained by God. Among etiological factors, food was mentioned five times, a blow on the head five times, heredity five times, worries or thinking too much four times, study four times, syphilis three times, alcohol twice, poverty twice, and lack of sleep once. Here are the responses, beginning with those that emphasize disturbances of the head:

> Attendant Alfaro: As far as mental illness goes, it seems to me that so many people come to the Hospital and don't notice when one talks to them. If one asks them something, they say that they are in good condition. They don't notice anything. They have a disturbance in their heads. Mental illness comes from the head, bad feeding, or suffering from thinking that they are poor, that they will not have enough to take care of their small children. Disturbance has to come from that.

> Attendant Costa: Mental illnesses come from many causes. Sometimes they come from a blow on the head that one suffers, or other times they are hereditary. They can also come from

complications from other illnesses like syphilis or epilepsy.

Attendant Chacón: It can be a disturbance resulting from one's thoughts, or worries, or from liquor or insufficient food.

Attendant Durán: It's when one is disconcerted in one's ideas. It comes from too much studying and certain thoughts.

Attendant Fuentes: So what would it be? It's a sickness that disturbs one, one who is the patient who suffers from that sickness. They aren't responsible for their persons to anyone. It comes from the head. It's a weakness.

Attendant Ibáñez: It comes from too many ideas, too much thinking that disturbs the head. There's a change of ideas, when one thinks one thing on one side and on the other one thinks of one's family. There's a confusion of ideas. It comes from the worry one has about one's home. It comes from too many ideas that one has, too much thinking. And sometimes there isn't enough food. That's the way it seems to me.

Attendant Jiménez: It's when a person lacks understanding and suffers head disturbances. It comes from the head. There are many patients who can change their ideas.

Attendant León: I can't tell you. In some people it comes from too much thinking, and also if someone has suffered a blow to the head in an accident.

Attendant Llona: Mental illness is the change in real ideas to others that are outside our vocabulary. Mental illness makes a patient say things which are not to be understood. Such words come when the head isn't functioning well, so that the patient is not thinking about what he's saying.

Attendant Nores: It must be because there's a cerebral waste, or because people are nervous. They may suffer a nervous shock. Or they suffer a lot because they're not sleeping. It's a weakness in the head. It can also be from inheritance from sick parents.

Attendant Ortiz: It's a disturbance that one has in one's mind, and one doesn't realize it. It can come from birth, or also from a blow to the head. Also from inheritance from relatives, or sometimes from insufficient food that people have at home. There are times when they don't have enough food. Or from too much studying.

Attendant Paredes: Sometimes it comes from thinking. Other times it attacks the nerves. Sometimes from not eating or from studying.

The responses which focus on some loss of function are the following:

Attendant Bravo: It's the loss of an individual's knowing. Sometimes it's hereditary. And sometimes, who knows?

Attendant García: Mental illness is when a man loses understanding. It can come if one is not well fed during childhood. It often comes from studying. Syphilis is another cause.

Attendant Hoyos: It's a sickness where one frankly loses one's memory. It can be from a blow, or it's hereditary, or it comes from syphilis. I don't know any more about what it comes from.

Attendant Meza: It's when one loses all one's reason. A person doesn't know what he's doing or what he's going to do. It's outside ideas. It comes from the moment that they lose their understanding. Then they stop being normal.

And the response which refers to God is this one:

Attendant Estrada: There are some who take their time to get better and others who improve rapidly. Mental illness comes from not sleeping enough ["*malas noches*"] or drunkenness. Sometimes it's from women and others it comes from thinking about some property or other. And there are times when God ordains that sickness.

The Patients

Interviews were held with twenty-six patients, all of them men in Pavilion 20 as has been indicated. Overwhelmingly, the variable which allows the classification of responses to the question about mental illness is a matter, not of the subject's origins in demographic or ethnic terms, nor of his degree of education, but of the very character of his illness, a discovery which naively I did not anticipate. Thus, it is possible to group the responses, one one hand, of patients diagnosed as manic-depressive, alcoholic, or some other syndrome, and those with a diagnosis of schizophrenia, the first giving, with some exceptions which reflect the nature of the illness, adequate or more than adequate statements, and the second giving, with some exceptions which reflect their self-understanding, statements which tend toward inappropriate brevity, or even which negate or reject the question. The first grouping includes the following responses:

> Patient Aguila (manic-depressive, mania): For me it's the loss of psychic control which everyone has both in his private life and in his social life. What else can I tell you? It's difficult to describe. Usually it appears with insomnia and no appetite. Then there is a bad mood. There are special terms which I don't remember clearly. There are special symptoms: retreat in social life. It's a decay. There are endogenous and exogenous causes. What's inside one, the hereditary factor, for example. Then there are lesions which come with sicknesses like syphilis. Also malnutrition or ignorance of moral forces. There are persons who allow themselves to be beaten by disagreeable happenings. That is in regard to what one has inside oneself. In the environment there are socially unadaptable persons who carry with them a series of complexes that, to begin with, weaken their spiritual state, later turn into cases of definite illness that require the intervention of doctors.
>
> Patient Borja (reactive anxious depression): It is a psychic abnormality, nothing more. I couldn't define those things because I don't know about them.
>
> Patient Cabral (abnormal psychopathic personality, symptomatic alcoholism): If I understand you, the patient comes from outside to consult with the doctor, which is what he has to do to get cured. The doctor will say the rest according to the sickness he finds. If it's very urgent, the doctor, it seems to me, would advise him to get admitted immediately. On the other hand, if it's not very serious, to have outpatient treatment. It's according to how serious it is, according to the case he finds. How does it come? It can be from a chance accident. It can be from the abuse of one's health. It can be from some sexual abuse, a big nervous shock. And it comes from masturbation. Also from excesses in drinking alcohol.
>
> Patient Chocano (chronic alcoholism, alcoholic psychosis): We believe that it is one of the most difficult and complex illnesses that

science has to deal with, because in each case different states appear which psychiatry can explain. However, I repeat, each day terrain is being conquered in this field. The patient does not notice when he becomes ill and, generally, he believes that he himself is healthy. But this is observed only by one who really has not become ill. It could be said that the causes or origins are many. In some cases, with the schizophrenics, we can specify the origin or the causes when the disturbance is over soon. In other cases it's impossible. The psychiatrist is the one who decides.

Patient Dejo (manic-depressive, manic): It is an illness where one is disturbed and does not know what one is doing. One's nerves are attacked. I don't know how it comes. The nerves would be in the head. It also comes from insomnia, from worries.

Patient Ortiz (Manic-depressive, manic): It's one of the illnesses which exists in all the countries of the world. It comes from thinking too much. Sometimes from alcoholic parents or the lack of good food.

Patient Yáñez (psychomotor epilepsy): One moves on to a psychiatrist after being treated by a physician. The physician would specify what kind of a person one would be.

Patient Zevallos (manic-depressive, circular form): It's related to the head which is upset. It makes one do things one wouldn't do if one were in a good state of health. It's one's own fault if one has excesses or vices, some wickedness, if one has bad habits.

The schizophrenic patients responded this way:

Patient Estrada (paranoid schizophrenia): It's a sickness of the head and the nerves, just that. It comes with restlessness, anguish, and nervous agitation. It's hard to say. The doctors know about it. There are many reasons for it. In some it comes from physical blows and in others by moral blows.

Patient Flores (paranoid schizophrenia, paranoid): It comes from pressure, a suggestion from an idea that no matter how hard one tries one can't get rid of it. It's a penetrating idea, and one can't stop thinking about it in spite of how hard one tries to do it. So it's an idea that almost always doesn't become real. There are thoughts that torture a person. Often it's vulgar, in a word, from the people, the crowd. At the beginning they made me Christ. I screamed obscenities and other crazy things like that. I don't give any credit to those thoughts. It was a moral obsession.

Patient Gálvez (paranoid schizophrenia): It's a nervous crisis where the person has a variety of thoughts which don't come to constitute an idea in one's freedom to think. To begin with, it's that one has to forget about oneself. One lets go of morals, the qualities which exist in different senses. It varies according to the order and material for rubbing that it has for becoming manifest to the people who are close to the mental patient. For example, they are asking how to subdue one's health in order to show one's condition in advance. With the same idea, it is necessary to observe in order to realize what one has done or to take up a good action toward what has common sense, so that one comes to destroy the same sentiments for the same reason. It is always the same details which come to conquer a group in captivity to which right is denied. We say in this case that both the good and bad elements come together in quotes. They come together for the underblind and give a bit of good will for working or for expression.[3]

Patient Huerta (paranoid schizophrenia): It's a sickness of the nervous system of the head. It has millions of organs and as many sicknesses. It happened to me for the first time because of my little girl's sickness. It's like any other sickness which happens in the body. It's from the organism.

Patient Iglesias (paranoid schizophrenia): It's a craziness. I don't know how it comes. It's from the nerves.

Patient Justo (paranoid schizophrenia): It's the atrophy of both mental and spiritual faculties which impede the carrying out of cerebral functions as they ought to be done, leading us, we may say like this, to lose the path. That's what I think. It can come by physical or somatic inheritance or it can be caught from others in different ways. In regard to physical or somatic inheritance, if one is the child of a demented father or mother. In regard to different causes, it can come from some blow to the head or some frustrated intention, some desire repressed involuntarily, or because of some misfortune.

Patient Lora (paranoid schizophrenia, paranoid): Man has his soul which is being developed in normal and abnormal life. It's from inheritance, ambition, environment. Sometimes some disturbance, an abnormal thing exists, which places a person under the necessity for a guide for the better development of reasoning. When it's not normal and one needs that guide, then the patient is mental. It comes from inheritance, or in my case guilt. It's the doctors' job, their obligation.

Patient Llerena (paranoid schizophrenia): It seems that somebody has said that it is a most surprising case for the beings to whom it comes.

Patient Márquez (catatonic schizophrenia): It's a sickness from not having been born well, from a person's not having been cared for.

Patient Negrín (paranoid schizophrenia): It seems to me that it's giving predominance to the imagination. Imaginitive things predominate. One dreams. One disengages too. In my case, to begin with, I had headaches. It comes from disorders in the organism. There are psychic forces inside one that influence one's understanding.

Patient Ñeco (paranoid schizophrenia): It's forgetting, what's called amnesia. It's forgetting everything, not remembering anything of what may have happened. It always comes from vices, always from being with women, drunkenness, being too studious.

Patient Peña (catatonic-hebephrenic schizophrenia): It's when people aren't with their heads in good order. They are bothered.

Patient Quintana (catatonic-paranoid schizophrenia): It's a disequilibrated disturbance of the head, a headache. It's crazy people, a crazy sickness. It comes from contagion from so many patients.

Patient Reyes (paranoid schizophrenia): I can't give a definition.

Patient Salas (paranoid schizophrenia): It's when occupations are useless and involuntary. That's all.

Patient Tapia (catatonic-paranoid schizophrenia): It happens from thinking. There are different ideas which occur in the mind, and in that way one begins to conjecture various things which aren't true. It comes from the bad thoughts that come to one.

Patient Ureta (paranoid schizophrenia): I don't have it. I'm not a mental patient.

Patient Vega (paranoid schizophrenia): It's when one feels incapable of of doing a thing one is asked to do, something a little difficult to do. One can't carry it out. It comes from some suffering, or when one works too much or studies too much. One can be affected with some mental illness.

An attempted correlation

On beginning the analysis of the data it was hypothesized that there would be a correlation of the responses to the questions about the ideology of mental illness and other responses to other questions in the schedule. For example, it was anticipated that the subjects who responded with organic concepts to the question which sought a definition of mental illnes would also offer responses that were more custodial[4] and authoritarian to the question, "What is the patient's duty?" (asked only of the psychiatrists, nurses, and aides). This was not the case. There was an overwhelming majority of all the categories asked who responded by emphasizing concepts like "obedience," "cooperation," or "good behavior," and very few respondents who offered any other kind of response. Among the twelve psychiatrists interviewed, Dr. Bueno, who gave an organic definition of mental illness, described his conception of the patient's duty as: "To cooperate with the doctor, accepting the therapy that is prescribed, communicating what he feels and everything that happens in relation to his person. To treat the nurses and aides well. This refers to the more agreeable and peaceful patients. The fact is that the patient in a state of agitation can't do that." In contrast, those who provided socio-psychological definitions of mental illness said the following about the patient's duty:

Dr. Alba: Depending on the type of patient, it's accepting the doctors' efforts to help him.

Dr. Espinoza: The primary duty for the patient is to obey all the orders given by the doctor. Then the patient himself has as his duty to report punctually on the service when leave is given to him, and to give information about the names of his relatives so that they can be contacted.

> Dr. López: He should have confidence in the doctor, follow instructions, and lend every possible effort to the progress of our medical knowledge, provided that this does not affect his health and comfort.

Nevertheless, some psychiatrists rejected the application of the notion of "duty" to the patient: Dr. Caso, who offered a psychological definition of mental illness, said: "In the first place, most of them don't believe they are patients. The patient should cooperate in any way possible, but he has his limitations from the illness itself. One of the symptoms can be the lack of cooperation, so one can't ask for cooperation as his duty because he is sincere." And Dr. Díaz offered: "There are so many kinds of patients that it is a difficult question. I don't believe they have to have a duty, but rather a great spirit of collaboration in order to secure their cooperation."

Of the thirteen nurses, only one, Nurse Esquivel, said that the patient had no duties: "The question isn't clear. It has to do with what is scheduled. He has to eat and go to bed at the right times, and to be at the nurse's orders for any contingency that can occur. One can't ask a patient in serious condition to have an obligation or a duty." It may be pointed out, however, that Nurse Esquivel made his statement to be conditional on the state of the patient. The other nurses gave responses that were clearly custodial-authoritarian. Nine defined the patient's duty in terms of "obeying," "accepting treatment," or "following orders," as represented in the following examples:

> Nurse Bustos: Letting himself be treated.

> Nurse Frías: Being reachable or being obedient for his treatment.

> Nurse Hurtado: He should obediently follow all the doctor's orders, as carried out by the nurse.

And three nurses defined the patient's duty in terms of respect, as for examples:

> Nurse Chivas: He should have respect for the personnel. All the patients have to respect the white coat when they see it. They have to obey and cooperate.

> Nurse Lozada: Respecting and obeying staff orders.

Fourteen of the seventeen attendants, all of whom gave rather widely varied responses in regard to mental illness, defined the patient's duty in custodial-authoritarian terms:

> Attendant Alfaro: Above all, being at the orders of the aide, being obedient, and not being aggressive. The aide can't do favors for them if they don't behave well. So if they are good, the aide has the right to take good care of them.
>
> Attendant Costa: It's behaving themselves with the aides.
>
> Attendant Hoyos: Being good and respecting the nurses and the aides, and especially the doctors.
>
> Attendant Nores: It would be obeying what they are told to do. Taking their pills when the nurse tells them to, and eating their food.

The three exceptions gave other responses:

> Attendant Bravo: They don't have duties. Only the lucid ones have duties and can do their duty.
>
> Attendant Estrada: They should look to the aide and not hit another patient. Some of them are very good. They help out.
>
> Attendant Ibáñez: It seems to me that a patient doesn't have a duty. The way it is, one can't improve anything. Only the doctors make decisions.

Conclusion

Although the character of the sample, which is neither representative nor random, places limitations on the interpretation of the data--and in this manner we may draw out suggestions rather than conclusions--it is clear that there is a great variety of responses to the question which was intended to explore the ideology of mental illness. This is true for each one of the population categories of the Hospital. Beyond this, it appears that variation is even wider from one population category to another; and this shows a sharp division of points of view within the Hospital. The psychiatrists, clinical psychologists, and social workers, conditioned by their training and experience in their practice, gave responses which were formed more by theoretical considerations. It also appears that these professional persons were the ones with the greatest interest in therapeutic approaches to the treatment of mental patients. Thus, it can be said that concepts of mental illness were better informed, more therapeutic, and lead to more active intervention at the higher levels of Hospital structure; and they were less informed, more custodial, and more passive on the lower levels. There was a gap, then, between the elite of the hospital and the other categories of the population studied. Perhaps the role of the nurse, a person who was conditioned as much by his or her social origins in the popular strata as by training and supervisory position in the pavilion,[5] was more narrowly directed in the authoritarian-custodial direction, at least in the nurses' responses to the question. The patients and attendants, who constitute the largest parts of the Hospital population, were even farther separated from the elite than the nurses in their conceptions about mental illness. The attendants, for whom there existed no expectation of a therapeutic role (Stein 1963a:211), were ideologically segregated. One can say that they were almost completely excluded from any therapeutic functions the Hospital had, although my observations revealed many therapeutic actions and reactions on their part which occurred in their human relations with patients.[6] In the case of the patients, who generally offered highly personalized concepts of mental illness, it is possible that they had absorbed, in a less deliberate selse, or learned, more deliberately, some aspects of mental illness ideology from the other social categories of the Hospital, but it also appears that they would have done this largely through their contacts with other patients in conversations in the pavilion, because for the most part they do not reflect the ideologies of the Hospital elite.[7]

I am writing here of the pavilion structure that existed in 1959. Psychiatric facilities, as has been indicated at the outset, have evolved in Peru since then,[8] but it may be useful to record my feeling that this kind of range in conceiving mental illness in the total population of a psychiatric facility is contraindicated in any other type of institution than the traditional custodial one. That is to say, to the extent that the function of a psychiatric facility is therapeutic, the exclusion of some category or categories of personnel, especially the majority part or parts, from the understanding the elite have of their own conceptual instruments and purposes constitutes a serious dysfunction. At the very least, it is an obstacle for the pursuit of any therapeutic function. This applies, equally well, to the patients who appeared to be excluded also from such understanding, although, indeed, many of them are perforce excluded by the character of their own disorders. This may be a psychiatric problem, despite the very strong possibility that it is not encouraged by the psychiatrists: Kleinman (1980:113-114) speaks of the "cognitive distance" between doctor and patient as "an indicator of the clinician's ability to translate from an esoteric theoretical idiom to an idiom accessible to laymen."[9] In the case of the doctor-patient relationship, as has been noted, in a psychiatric hospital the nature of the illness also conditions cognitive distance. Here and elsewhere in the Hospital Hospital cognitive distances are evident both between and within sectors of the population. They may be viewed as constituting barriers to the therapeutic processes which are the foundations of its existence.

Notes

1. Unconscious because while the Hospital's people understood well that the different social strata held ideas which were different from each other, nobody in the upper strata was aware that the lower strata were *excluded* from information.

2. All the names of those interviewed are disguised. I have assigned fictitious names to them alphabetically, according to the order of the interviews.

3. I do not guarantee this translation from the Spanish. In some ways it may come close to Patient Gálvez's intent; but in other ways it may merely parallel his intent.

4. "Custodialism" (see Stein and Oetting 1964) refers to a traditional concept of the mental hospital and its functioning. It places emphasis on authority, security, and protection. It accompanies organic ideologies of mental illness, in contrast with "humanism" which focuses on therapeutic optimism and socio-psychological ideologies.

5. In this it appears that the Peruvian nurse resembles North American and British nurses, according to M. Jones (1962:62) who observes that although the latter have a higher status than the attendants "and a professional image which implies knowledge which frequently [they] do not possess . . . [they] may have had no formal training in psychiatry other than a short affiliation as [students]. Most R. N.'s have been trained in a fairly strict, authoritarian culture." In their role within the nursing unit also, M. Jones (1953:38) points out in his well known earlier contribution on the "therapeutic community," the nurse relates to the group as a whole and "does not participate in a psychotherapeutic relationship with a single patient."

6. Colarelli and Siegel (1966), in their research on the development of paraprofessionals among the aides of Topeka State Hospital, show very effectively that the aide can indeed take a therapeutic role within a psychiatric service--even if the fiscal arrangements of the institution do not permit adequate compensation for aides who are doing more work and more creative work.
7. Here, too, it seems that there exists great unrealized potential for the integration of patients into a "therapeutic community." See M. Jones (1953).
8. As a good indication of such development, Arnillas Arana, Otárola, et al. (1970:388) report on an experiment with a therapeutic community in Pavilion 6 of the same Hospital Víctor Larco Herrera, one which involved a team of psychiatrists, nurses, social workers, one psychologist, a nursing assistant, the pavilion aides, and a representative of the patients in which "hierarchies were abolished, giving complete autonomy to the Community." Innovations were instituted, such as "daily group meetings of an instructional type, readings, sports, occupational therapy, dances," and other gatherings. These researchers conclude that such an effort "has produced positive results, really surprising ones in some clinical cases: great progress in resocialization, optimal motivation of personnel, considerable material achievement to the benefit of Pavilion 6 and of the patients, notable reduction of personal conflicts among the patients, impressive limitation of the use of medications, and good prospects for the future."
9. Kleinman (1980:104-105) suggests an "explanatory model" framework," consisting of "the notions about an episode of sickness and its treatment that are employed by all those engaged in the clinical process." Such models "are held by patients and practitioners in all health care systems." He (ibid.:115) adds that this framework "suggests that there are now ways to evaluate the quality and success of at least one clinical task: communication with patients."

Chapter 3

What is a Mental Hospital?

I

In this Chapter I deal with the two faces of a mental hospital: one, that of treatment, medical and moral therapy, and assistance for troubled human beings; the other, that of incarceration, coercion, and segregation. While the personnel of such a hospital may articulate therapeutic goals, and may believe sincerely in these, there also exist structures which contradict what they articulate and believe. Thus, the mental hospital contains a contradiction. I would like to refer to this contradiction as *structural ambivalence*, taking as my model the attraction-repulsion, love-hate, affirmation-denial characteristic of the human psyche but applying it to the structure of an institution rather than that of a person. What I am trying to do here is to approach a collective, or corporate, self-concept comparable to the "situated knowlege" with three components, defined by to Rhodes (1991:174) in her study of an emergency psychiatric unit:

> The first [component] was the knowledge of how to situate the

> "knowledge of medicine" within the reality of practice. . . . The second . . . was their resistance to the knowledge of medicine and the discipline of the unit. This resistance was oblique, not opposed as "truth" to some sort of singular oppressive power, but developed at an angle to the expected definitions of situations. The staff were cunning, devious, and actively ignorant in moving among the threads of power on the unit, taking advantage of areas of invisibility. . . . Finally, the staff's situated knowledge included a self-conscious awareness that it *was* a situated knowledge. Mostly spoken, subject to changes of all kinds, it was recognized by them to be homemade and fragile. They urged me to write it down partly, I think, for that reason.

The same goal is sought, in a less complicated and technical way, by Allderidge (1985:19) in her historical study of "Bedlam," the popular name for Bethlem Hospital:

> Bethlem--or rather its custodians--did not pretend to offer either refuge, good care or cure. "Good care" I shall leave aside, because we are talking about what the custodians pretended to offer, not what we think of what they did offer, and I do not myself know enough of what went on in their minds to speak for them. This is a pefectly serious point, because there is plenty of scope for research into what the governors of Bethlem, and others similarly placed at other institutions, really did think they were providing in the way of care. Unless we accept that they were all very uncomplicated sadistic monsters, which I see no reason to accept, then their doubtless multifarious views on what they thought they were doing must surely have some relevance in the history of psychiatry.

What do the custodians of madness think they are doing? And what do they really do? It is the discrepancy that we are after. As Rapoport (1960:11) points out, we have learned from studies of mental hospitals "that communication channels and processes have a relevance for patient care; that the structure of authority relations is relevant; that social processes occur that are unknown to the staff or undesired by them, but which cannot be overlooked if the *real* rather than the *ideal* social situation is to be coped with; and that any patient is involved in a network of rlationships each of which has some influence on his emotional life and behavior." York (1955:261-262) says in his study of a veterans' mental hospital near Boston, "it should be recalled that the social attitudes and practices prevailing at any one time are generally accepted uncritically with little awareness of the degree to which they may limit creativity in ideas or spontaneity in action. Just as years hence we shall find that many now favored practices were barriers to patient welfare and staff efficiency, . . . we need to bear in mind that [the hospital] sincerely believed it was striving to give the best care available to patients."

This is a social anthropological, rather than a clinical, study of iatrogenesis. It aims to describe the antitherapeutic face of psychiatric patient care, an aspect of a hospital that its staff may be completely unaware of. Thus, no one may know that the hospital exists at cross-purposes with itself. The data that will be used to illustrate this structural ambivalence originate in a Peruvian mental hospital which clearly showed me its different faces.

II

According to Goffman (1962:4-5), mental hospitals are included among five types of "total institutions": those "established to care for persons felt to be both incapable and harmless," e.g., "the blind, the aged, the orphaned, and the indigent"; those "for persons felt to be both incapable of looking after themselves and a threat to the community," e.g., tubercular cases, mental patients, and lepers; those "organized to protect the community against what are felt to be intentional dangers to it," e.g., criminals, prisoners of war, and inhabitants of concentration camps; those organized for some specific job, e.g., army posts, ships, residential schools, work camps, and colonial quarters; and those "designed as retreats from the world," e.g., "abbeys, monasteries, convents, and other cloisters." Goffman (ibid.:203) summarizes the features of such establishments:

> Institutions like mental hospitals are of the "total" kind, in the sense that the inmate lives all of the aspects of his life on the premises in the close company of others who are similarly cut off from the wider world. These institutions tend to contain two broad and quite differently situated categories of participants, staff and inmates, and it is convenient to consider the secondary adjustments of the two categories separately.

It should be remembered, however, as Etzioni (1970:138) notes, that the mental hospital is usually a total institution only for the patients; and this was the case in the hospital in Lima, Peru, since both medical and paramedical personnel neither lived nor had all their social contacts exclusively within it, but had their families, friends, other work activities, professional or union associations, and even their greater aspirations centered in their lives outside.[1]

There exists a continuing debate[2] on the character, goals, effects, and social utility of mental hospitals, whether they are good or bad, whether they alleviate pain or cause it, and whether they cure mental illness or make it worse. Dwyer (1987:1) traces this to the last century:

> During the nineteenth century, insane asylums were simultaneously scourged as "tombs of the living dead" and praised as loving places of refuge to which troubled Americans could retreat for comfort and care. Such controversy over the functions of these institutions, and the meaning of their history, has persisted into the twentieth century, reviving with particular intensity in the 1960s and 1970s.

Grob (1979:135-136) says:

> Anyone concerned with the development of mental hospitals . . . immediately confronts a scholarly controversy. On one side stand those who celebrate these institutions as evidence of human progress, humanitarianism, and liberal sentiment. Although these scholars concede that there are serious flaws and imperfections in these institutions, they operate on the assumption that with additional effort and funding, most societal defects could have been eliminated. On the other, there are those scholars who denigrate these same institutions, viewing them as the agencies by which dominant elites restrained deviant groups, or largely lower class elements, thereby ensuring their own hegemony.

Levinson and Gallagher (1964:14) define institutions for the care of the mentally ill in terms of four functions: the "incarcerative function," to protect the community from individuals "considered involuntarily dangerous due to 'illness'"; the "life-maintaining function," to protect patients "from their own self-destructive impulses"; the "care function," to maintain the patient "during the period when he [sic] is judged unresponsible"; and the "therapeutic-rehabilitative function," to intervene in order to help the patient "reduce his vulnerabilities and develop his inner resources so he can again pursue his life course in society." Scull (1979:173), speaking of British asylums of the nineteenth century, but with relevance to many of today's custodial institutions, says that, "by sustaining the illusion that asylums were medical institutions, they placed a humanitarian and scientific gloss on the community's behaviour, legitimizing the removal of difficult and troublesome people whose confinement would have been awkward to justify on other grounds." In discussing the "formative period of asylumdom," early in the last century, Mellett (1982:163-164) similarly notes the "dual purpose" of the institution: "the protection of the community against individuals who apparently constituted a threat to its security, and the provision of a therapeutic milieu, or at least humane custodial care, for the labelled insane," which "meant that from the beginning, the institution had an ambivalent character, with potentially conflicting responsibilities: to the community and to the patient." Scull (1993:141) shows how "a pathological environment . . . encourages the very behaviors which are then used to justify its existence"; while "some inmates manage to adjust to them . . . it is one of the ironies of institutional existence that those who manage this transition most effectively are at the same time reducing their ability to function in the outside world." Chamberlin (1978:6), an ex-mental patient, asserts that the structure of the mental hospital is anti-therapeutic:

> People who are labeled mentally ill become part of a system that deprives them of control over their own life as part of their treatment. Mental hospitals have been called 'total institutions', in which even such ordinary decisions as when to eat, go to the toilet, and go to bed are made by others. A natural consequence of being subjected to such a regimen is a feeling of depersonalization. Feelings of depersonalization are frequently considered primary symptoms of mental illness. To complete the circle, psychiatrists usually attribute their patients' feelings of depersonalization to their internal state and not to conditions within mental institutions.
>
> The whole experience of mental hospitalization promotes weakness and dependency. Not only are the lives of patients controlled, but patients are constantly told that such control is for their own good, which they are unable to see because of their mental illness. Patients become unable to trust their own judgment, become indecisive, overly submissive to authority, frightened of the outside world. The antitherapeutic nature of mental hospitaliztion has long been recognized.

Bockoven (1972:1-2) begins his study of community psychiatric facilities with the question, "What is a mental hospital?", and adds this statement:

> The typical mental hospital impresses a visitor approaching its grounds as having something of the appealing quality of a college campus, with the exception that there are almost no people passing to and fro on the walks. . . . It is not until one enters the wards where the patients live that one feels the impact of what it means to be a patient. . . . Contrary to one's expectations, ward after ward may be passed through without witnessing the violent, the grotesque, or the ridiculous. Instead, one absorbs the heavy atmosphere of hundreds of people doing nothing and showing interest in nothing. Endless lines of people sit on benches along the walls. Some have their eyes closed; others gaze fixedly at the floor or the opposite wall. Occasionally, a head is turned to look out a window or to watch someone coming back from the toilet to take his place on a bench. All in all, it is a scene of inertness, listlessness, docility and hopelessness. . . . The visitor finds that the scene . . . appalls him with the emptiness and pointlessness of human life. . . . He must strain his imagination to see how the surrender of actually thousands of people to abject despair and inertia could possibly represent an improvement in their mental condition. On the contrary, he can envision himself going out of his mind if forced to spend many days in such a setting.

With more kindness, yet in recognition that such institutions are still imperfect, Haugsgjerd (1980:203-204) says:

> What is a mental hospital? . . . . If we start from our best intentions, we could perhaps say, as some colleagues have done, that the mental hospital should be some kind of a university, where people who have to, can learn something that cannot be learnt otherwise: about regressions, about anxieties, about how to restitute a world to live in after you have experienced a catastrophic collapse in your psyche. The realities, however, are almost always a far cry from these intentions. . . . The mental hospital is therefore more properly described as a site where immense deposits of mental pain can be found.

And Braginsky, Braginsky, and Ring (1969:216) report one mental patient's response to their question, "What is the hospital supposed to do, in your opinion?":

> Several things. It depends on what's wrong with you. If all you need to do is get away from somebody that's bothering you, this is a very fine place to go. And then this place is maybe just a custodial place--you can't take care of yourself, so you let other people get you up, make sure you get dressed, go to meals. And then it's a place you can go when you want to get away from all stress, you want to hide from the world, and, in being this way, you're still acceptable to some people--like people here. Again, it doesn't make any difference what you do down here; it's expected that you should act crazy because you are. It's a haven. But I guess for some people it's a place to get some sort of help. Supposed to get some people to understand yourself, how to cope with life and all that.

Mental hospitals have a relatively short history. Martini P. (1983:16) points out:

> In classical times, the "madman" did not have an autonomous status. His or her public behaviors were assimilated into the wide territory of "non-reason", a position shared with "witches", beggars, prostitutes, delinquents, those afflicted with neurological disorders, and so forth. No specific place existed for the "mentally ill," except for a generalized seclusion space which made them like other figures which, by their behavior or by their social role, were marginal to the economic structure and the dominant values belonging to preindustrial societies.

Thus, in the beginning there were only those marginal persons, the insane, those suffering from physical illnesses, vagabonds, beggars, and other poor people. In those times, according to Parry-Jones (1972:6-7), no separate provisions for the insane were made and harmless lunatics and idiots continued to be left at liberty as long as they were not considered to be dangerous. They were taken care of in the hospitals of the medieval era; and even in the seventeenth century in England there were no separate institutions for the mentally ill, but "harmless lunatics and idiots continued to be left at liberty as long as they were not considered to be dangerous and caused no social disturbance." Until the end of the eighteenth century, Foucault (1965:65) says, only one-tenth of the inmates of the Hôpital Général in Paris were mad. K. Jones (19551-2) says of eighteenth-century England:

> There was no clear definition of what constituted insanity, and certainly no recognition of the insane as a separate social class

> requiring a distinct form of treatment. The problem was a submerged one. Only a small proportion of the total number were recognized as being insane, and the majority were treated as though they were fully responsible for their actions. If their mental condition reduced them to penury, they came within the purview of the Poor Law. If it led them to break the criminal code, they were judged by the penal law. If they wandered abroad from their legal place of settlement without means of support, they were involved in the rigours of the vagrancy laws.

In England there was one exception, according to Porter (1987a:122-123), the Priory of the Order of St. Mary of Bethlehem, known also as "Bethlem" or "Bedlam," a receptacle for lunatics after 1377 and, in the eighteenth century a freakshow for the entertainment of Londoners: "It was traditionally a favorite resort for sightseers. Until around 1770 they simply turned up, Sundays excepted, being expected to drop some coppers into the poor box . . . . Spectators thronged to see the unaccommodated man. And largely because Bethlem housed the only collection of mad-people in the nation, it achieved a sort of concentrated notoriety; it became an epitome of all that people fantasized about madness itself." In the early decades of nineteenth century United States, similarly, the insane provided a source of amusement: Dain (1964:51) notes how "Crowds still flocked to the Pennsylvania Hospital on Sundays . . . to amuse themselves by teasing the inmates and watching their antics. There was a small fee for this questionable pleasure."

McGovern (1985:15) observes that the historical precondition for the existence of asylums for the mad was when "madness became threatening rather than harmless, and the mad suffered loss of liberty as communities increasingly confined them on poor farms or in almshouses or jails." Scull (1979:13-14) notes:

> The typical response to the deranged underwent dramatic changes in English society between the mid-eighteenth and mid-nineteenth centuries. At the outset of this period, mad people for the most part were not treated even as a separate category or type of deviants. Rather, they were assimilated into the much larger, more amorphous class of the morally disreputable, the poor, and the impotent, a group which also included vagrants, minor criminals, and the physically handicapped. Furthermore, just as in the case of the indigent generally, the societal response to the problems posed by the presence

of mentally disturbed individuals did not involve segregating them into separate receptacles designed to keep them apart from the rest of society. The overwhelming majority of the insane were still to be found at large in the community. By the mid-nineteenth century, however, virtually no aspect of this traditional response remained intact. The insane were clearly and sharply distinguished from other "problem populations." They found themselves incarcerated in a specialized, bureaucratically organized, state-supported asylum system which isolated them both physically and symbolically from the larger society.

III

The evolution of Peruvian psychiatry followed the same course of movements elsewhere in the world. A reading of Valdizán (1988), on treatment of the mad during colonial times, or Valdivia Ponce (1989), on the history of Peruvian psychiatry, affirms this view. Valdizán includes some cases apparently from beyond the limits of psychiatry, but in his parade of disturbed persons, many seem to fit well into the pathological categories of contemporary psychiatry, although it also seems that with some, as he says, "there existed a good dose of tolerance" in colonial society (Valdizán 1988:136). According to Valdivia Ponce (1989:23) data from the Viceroyalty reveal "obsessions, halucinations, delusionss and other psychopathological evidence of the mentally ill," although they were interpreted as "bewitchments, revelations, and demoniacal and divine possessions." Mariátegui (1987:257) says: "Mental illness in remote times was tied to the supernatural, the divine, and the sacred. Thus, as in classical mythology there existed deities who caused and protected mental illnesses, in the Western world Christian tradition allows us to identify certain saints related to the protection and cure of mental disturbances."

According to Mariátegui (1985a:12-13), the first hospital for mental patients was established in 1859. This service, the *Hospicio del Cercado* [Inner City Hospice or Poorhouse], "also called the *Manicomio* [Madhouse], House of the Insane, or Asylum of Mercy." This hospital, the same author (ibid.:9-11) notes, was the successor of the "madhouses" of earlier centuries, the Hospitals of Santa Ana, established in 1549 for women, and San Andrés, established in 1552 for men, which "had special sections available for mental patients." While Ruiz

Zevallos (1994:47) suggests that the "*manicomio* formed part of a whole repressive system, of which the point of departure was the controlist obsessions of the elites in power," he also notes that its opening was a response "to the concrete need to put an end to a relation to madness based solely on brutal treatment and seclusion" (ibid:31). Delgado (1992:97) describes the new Manicomio del Cercado:

> For its time it was a rather good asylum, but a very small one as it proved to be shortly afterward. . . . The equipment and arrangement of the Hospicio gives some idea of the methods of treatment in those times. It had surprise baths; baths for disturbed persons, like those in the Salpetrière; restraint chairs for the containment of the disturbed, made in Paris. (The Sisters of Charity later added the so called "*cujas*" ["buckets"], cages in which patients were shut up, with locks, from which they could not leave, or even sit down comfortably to eat.) The establishment had 4 sections: the first, for calm patients; the second, for patients who periodically became excited; the third, for idiots, epileptics, and dirty patients; and the fourth, eight cells for the furious.

Mariátegui (1985a:23) calls Hermilio Valdizán, a Peruvian psychiatrist[3] educated in Europe, "the founding figure of Peruvian psychiatry." Mariátegui (1988:65) indicates that in 1918 "the Sociedad de Beneficencia Pública de Lima [the Lima Public Charity Society] opened the Asilo Colonia de La Magdalena [Magdalena Plantation Asylum] . . . called after 1930 the Hospital Víctor Larco Herrera, in honor of its benefactor," Valdizán being appointed in 1919 as head resident physician. Mariátegui (1985b:5) adds that Valdizán and his colleagues reformed the latter asylum in the same year, acting "to retire the Sisters of Charity--poor bearers of that name--who came from the Manicomio del Cercado to occupy themselves with mental patients":

> The backward belief in illness as sin and of the mentally ill person as possessed by the devil, did not permit the scientific treatment of mental patients. Valdizán, as Resident Physician, saw himself as impotent to act in defense of the patients, who were subjected to cruel methods of restraint and tormenting coercive procedures.

Mariátegui (1990:31-32) elsewhere elaborates on the history of the Hospital:

> The inoperability of regulations and the limited functions of doctors in the Asylum was due to the influential perseverance of the Sisters of Charity who endeavored to continue in the new establishment the repressive and inhumane system--peculiar to their demonological and perverse conception of mental disorder--which was maintained for a long time in the old Hospicio del Cercado which was also in their charge. In a city like Lima, with its hypocritical religiosity, the need for the departure of the Sisters of Charity as a necessary step to reform and humanize care for the mental patients, created a difficult situation because of the protectionist attitude of "Lima society" and the distinguished directors of the Public Charity Society of Lima, the Asylum's proprietary entity. Without the intervention of Don Víctor Larco Herrera's tenacity and economic power, representing the wealthy agrarian bourgeoisie rising to power, the reform movement for the care of the insane in the country, which then lagged more than a century behind what was taking place in Europe, would have been held back even more. The assistance of a committed, influential, and rich layman allowed technical criteria to prevail over the weight of tradition and physicians to take over their proper functions completely.

This was the institution in which my research took place. For the purposes of this essay, I select some themes from my observations and interviews which deal with the images of a mental hospital that the inhabitants, the personnel and the patients, project. With an informal question schedule, I asked the several categories of the hospital population about their conceptions of a mental hospital. Only the doctors gave me rich and varied responses: the twelve who answered the question, "In your opinion what is a mental hospital?"[4], offered a balance between "mental" and "behavioral" images: For example, Dr. Alba said, "A mental hospital is a specialized part of medicine whose object is the study and treatment of behavioral disorders in their most varied expressions. And it includes complete research on mental disorders." Dr. Chávez: "A mental hospital is an institution where care is given to different mental disturbances, primarily in relation to the upsets that these sick people provoke in society or in their homes." Dr. Espinoza: "At least in our context a mental hospital is the place where attention is given to both acute and chronic patients, for persons who have episodes of their mental illnesses." Dr. Ibarra: "A mental hospital is an establishment dedicated to the treatment of insane patients and with that object it studies the sick person with multidimensional criteria, in order to carry out the most adequate therapy and try to place him or her in an optimal state of mental health, or to make it possible for him or her to live in society." In addition, I asked them about the goals of the pavilions in which they worked ("What is the goal of Pavilion [n]? What should it achieve?"), and this question helped greatly to widen this base of custody-therapy-rehabilitation, revealing additional concepts of research, teaching, and economization:

> Dr. Alba: It is the same as in all the pavilions. They all have the same goal, the study of the patient and his or her treatment. We can differentiate them because a chronic pavilion has more custodial care. Here we do more in active study and treatment to secure the patient's reintegration in the community with the best functioning of his personality.
>
> Dr. Bueno: For this pavilion the first consideration is that it should march in tune with universal therapy. It should be a support for the orientation of the other pavilions and it should serve as a model for other psychiatric hospitals which may be formed in our national territory. For that it needs all the conveniences of a modern psychiatric pavilion, that is, what is current.
>
> Dr. Caso: In a general sense it should give patients the best care possible, both in- and outpatients. There exist limitations to this care, for example, economic ones, for at times there are no medicines. Then personnel is another problem. It would be ideal to have a group of permanent attendants appointed. As for the doctors, there are a few students, but it isn't the same. Also, better stipends for the doctors.
>
> Dr. Chávez: The goal ought to be a single one. It should have the status of a clinic, of a neuropsychiatric research center. It should develop certain laws and principles in the field of psychiatry.
>
> Dr. Díaz: It is a clinic. All the patients pay. They send them from admission after they are given treatment. We also get insured people, both white- and blue-collar workers.[5] We get many older persons who are abandoned by their families.
>
> Dr. Espinoza: This pavilion was especially created for patients who can achieve a social remission and thus be reincorporated in their families.

Dr. Fernández: According to the ones who built it, it should serve as a receptacle for chronic patients. But this is neither desirable nor what current circumstances require. There are many mental patients, including acute cases, who ought to be admitted into the pavilion for their improvement, but this is hard to obtain because of the orientation hospital authorities have given to this pavilion. It is for chronic patients and this greatly limits the benefits which could be achieved if we had the freedom to admit or hospitalize those acute patients who urgently need isolation from their family circles and treatment. Currently we reluctantly carry out the imposed orientation and we look with much sympathy for the admission of patients by making personal requests, in which the Director [i.e., the Medical Director not the Administrator] of the hospital assists us. Unfortunately, the Director has little power. The outside authorities, those in the Benefit Society, make trouble.

Dr. Gómez: Its goal is to care for chronic and indigent patients. That is the goal of Pavilion [n]. They have received all the treatments and have not recuperated. They don't have the money for another kind of pavilion. So they come to [n].

Dr. Herrera: The objective of Pavilion [n] is to obtain the maximum attention and therapeutic return within the human and material possibilities it has available. It should be turned into a model clinic, for which greater economic means are needed.

Dr. Ibarra: The objective is the total or partial cure of patients and their reintegration in social life. It would be desirable for this labor to be the most complete and lasting possible.

Dr. Jara: The treatment of acute psychotic patients in general, with some chronic ones, with biological and psychotherapeutic methods, including occupational therapy.

Dr. López: It should perform three activities through the work of a team: carrying out treatment and social rehabilitation of the patient, education and teaching, and research.

The thirteen nurses and seventeen attendants I interviewed gave more stereotyped answers to the question, "What is a hospital like Víctor Larco Herrera?" Among the nurses, eleven said that it was "a hospital to take care of mental patients," "where mental patients were treated," or simply "for mental patients" or "for mental illnesses." Two gave other responses. Three typical statements are reproduced here:

> Nurse Cruz: It is a place for patients where they are given due medical and nursing care in order to relieve them, reestablish them and cure them of psychic and physiological disturbances. It also has research goals in order to be able to get a better idea of this branch of medicine which is still only partly developed because it doesn't know very deeply the causes of mental disturbances which are believed to be multiple.
>
> Nurse Delgado: It is a diagnostic hospital where all patients who have mild, acute, and chronic disturbances of the nervous system are treated.
>
> Nurse Hurtado: It is where patients who have lost their reason are treated.

Attendants' responses to the same question were parallel to these, with fourteen stating that the hospital was "psychiatric", "for mental patients", "for the treatment of mental patients", or simply "for patients". The three which are presented here said something different:

> Attendant Alfaro: It is a hospital like a house where there are all kinds of medicines to cure the sick person, to improve his situation.
>
> Attendant García: It belongs to the Lima Public Benefit Society to which it was donated by the person whose name it bears. A mental hospital has the goal of giving treatment to all the patients in Peru who require that treatment, and to place itself always in contact with psychiatric advances of neighboring countries.
>
> Attendant León: It's like a quality hospital.

More varied and revealing were the responses of the nurses to the questions, "What thing should Pavilion [n] (or this hospital) achieve? What is the goal, why does it exist?", and they deserve exposition in more detail:

> Nurse Arruga: This pavilion exists to cure patients. It is to be able to obtain the discharge of the greatest number possible.
>
> The hospital is for curing mental patients so that they can be incorporated into their ordinary lives.

Nurse Bustos: Here it has turned into a teaching center for psychiatry. The goal is to give the best instruction to students in the Faculty of Medicine.

The hospital exists to take care of mental patients.

Nurse Cruz: The goal of the pavilion is, now, to take care of patients so they can then leave cured or improved and not to be simply a place of asylum for those patients. Because then the pavilion would fill up with patients, and all that would rest in the hands of the nurses and the doctors.

The basic function of the hospital would be the treatment of mental patients. It is also a center for research in the specialty of psychiatry, because there are private clinics and sanatoriums which do not have this goal but rather a commercial one. We have seen that patients from such private places come here in the same condition, and that they leave here reestablished and content, as they themselves say.

Nurse Chivas: The pavilion has to have its conveniences. Here the pavilions are classified. This one is for general medicine.

The hospital is to shelter and cure mental patients. It's an asylum.

Nurse Delgado: The pavilion is to give a pleasant place for the patient so that he doesn't miss his home, and so that he feels stimulated and cooperates in his treatment.

The hospital is for giving the patient back his health, with those where there are possibilities for recuperation. And for isolating chronic patients from society.

Nurse Esquivel: Here the pavilion is for taking care of patients.

The hospital should take up a reform in accord with the times. it ought to give better care to more patients and give better working conditions to people who have to work here, the doctors, the nurses, and the attendants.

Nurse Frías: This pavilion is for instruction in psychiatry.

The hospital should offer everything that the service needs.

Nurse Godoy: The pavilion is for the wellfare of the patients.

The welfare of the hospital is also necesary. They should see to what each pavilion needs, especially all the medications. If the personnel didn't exist, the hospital wouldn't exist. They have to look after its whole team.

Nurse Hurtado: Here are found almost all the non-recuperable patients. This pavilion is a charity one. At the least it should provide the best atmosphere.

In the hospital, in the first place, they should improve the economic situation for its servants. And it should also offer its services to everyone so that all the patients can receive good treatment and good food.

Nurse Iglesias: The pavilion? I don't understand the question. What is in the hands of the hospital is the matter of being more vigilant to prevent the escape of the sick people.

Nurse Justo: In accord with the hospital's economy, this pavilion has what it needs.

The hospital ought to build new pavilions to make room for the many sick people who are walking around in the streets.

Nurse Lozada: Here a special department is needed for the patients' recreation.

The hospital needs more money to construct more pavilions.

Nurse Llosa: The pavilion needs libraries and places for recreation.

The hospital lacks a real social work service.

The attendants responded to the same two questions in ways that also revealed more intricate pictures:

Attendant Alfaro (only to the first question): This is a hospital for poor people who are detained here. It's so that their situation will improve. It's a hospital for their own good. Because it's such a big hospital, there are many very sick people. There isn't any other place for poor people. It's also so that the doctors and other people have a place to work, so that they can take care of the patients.

Attendant Bravo: The pavilion is for taking care of all the patients who need the doctor's attention. It is concerned with the quick recuperation of the patients.

The goal of the hospital is to protect all the patients who ask for it. It doesn't always depend on the administration but it's the Charity Society which doesn't have the funds to protect every person who needs it.

Attendant Costa: The pavilion exists to take in mental patients and give them treatment.

The hospital's goal is curing mental patients.

Attendant Chacón: The pavilion gives facilities for working. There are many things that keep an attendant [he uses the word *empleado* ("employee")[6]] from doing his work here. For example, every request one makes, for soap and other things, they don't give one in this pavilion. Many things are lacking: creosote, flit, and hygienic things that shouldn't be lacking here. There should be bathrooms for attendants, but such things don't exist here. In the smaller pavilions these things exist.

The hospital is the service center for all the pavilions.

Attendant Durán: The pavilion is so that the patients can recuperate, returning complete health to them.

The hospital exists to give the patients back their health, with the doctors' help, so that a lot of healthy people go out to the city to work.

Attendant Estrada: The pavilion is for the patients.

The hospital is for interning patients who are to be found on the streets or in their houses.

Attendant Fuentes: The other pavilions were full of patients. Since there wasn't any room they built Pavilion [n].

The hospital exists so that patients can be here, so that mental patients won't be walking around in the streets.

Attendant García: This pavilion exists to give treatment to the patients, both interned ones and outpatients.

The hospital is for curing mental patients.

Attendant Hoyos: This pavilion is for giving treatment to the patients who enter.

The hospital exists to treat patients.

Attendant Ibáñez: The pavilion ought to be clean and the patients ought to be in treatment. Because of that we see more patients coming in and going out.

The hospital should excel in having a patient come, get well, and leave. Then another one can come in. This would be the goal.

Attendant Jiménez: The goal of Pavilion [n] is so that all the necessary material can exist so that employees and patients can work together, that is, so that the employees can have all that they need to be able to work more easily, and for the doctors and nurses, too, so that they have what they need to do the work that has to be done.

The goal the hospital ought to attain is that it ought to have all the personnel necessary and also have good doctors who are skilled so that they can easily take on the treatment of mental patients. And it also ought to have all kinds of machines and instruments that are needed in a hospital like Víctor Larco Herrera which is for mental patients.

Attendant León: Pavilion [n] exists so that the patients will be comfortable, so they can be calm, because this is a comfortable pavilion.

Here we have people who don't pay, and the hospital is happy to have them. That isn't so in other hospitals. Some of the patients work and help, and others don't. The hospital is happy to take care of them.

Attendant Llona: The pavilion should have all its conveniences, so that water, for example, is not lacking. It should have more employees so that there can be more progress.

The hospital should make sure that all the pavilions have more medicine, so that all the patients who come in can go out healthy and go back to work.

Attendant Meza: Pavilion [n] exists to receive a lot of insured and paying patients, so that all the patients here can get back their health. Because most of them come without being aware of it, and only their relatives bother about it. They come seriously ill.

The goal of the hospital is to build enough pavilions, for both men and women. To improve things they would have to open one or two more, emergency rooms, because in reality only those with money and who can pay are admitted here. We need more.

Attendant Nores: Things should go well in the pavilion.

The hospital gives the patients the best comforts it can. They should improve the food.

Attendant Ortiz: The pavilion exists for the patients in it, just that.

The hospital exists for the mental patients that exist.

Attendant Paredes: In this pavilion there is outpatient service for

> the patients who have attacks. They bring them in from outside to take care of them. The services take care of all kinds of illnesses. And there are also interned patients.
>
> The hospital is for mental patients, to intern them so they won't be out in the streets. There are a lot of them out there.

It is quite clear in these excerpts from the interviews that all personnel, from the professionals to the attendants, think of the hospital and themselves as involved in therapy, curing, and the return of patients to their ordinary lives. The doctors, who need to relate themselves to the worldwide field of psychiatric medicine, and some nurses, emphasize certain professional goals like study, research, and teaching. Most of the nurses place more emphasis on the cure, welfare, and comfort of their patients; while the attendants focus on the interning, protection, and care of patients. All of them tend to reject the custodial function and prefer to seek identities that have to do with treatment, patient recuperation, and the return of patients to their homes, jobs, and society. Many responses, also, refer to the institutional functions[7] of improving economic and working conditions for personnel, or of extending the hospital with the construction of more facilities and the employment of more personnel. Thus the pavilions and the hospital appear to have an actively therapeutic atmosphere. It is difficult to find negative themes, apart from the economic restrictions imposed by the administration or the Charity Society. Nevertheless, the mental hospital has another face, much less in the sense of any deficiency in the personnel or in their motives but more in the sense of its very structure.

IV

Goffman (1962:363-364) observes that "since inappropriate behavior is typically behavior that someone does not like and finds extremely troublesome, decisions concerning it tend to be political, in the sense of expressing the special interests of some particular faction or person." This is the structure from which arises the incarcerative function of the madhouse. Some of the patients I interviewed recognized this fact: Patient Borja, for example, told me, "They mark you here. They took a picture of me. It's like being a prisoner"; and Patient Flores said, "This is a pavilion of prisoners, crazy persons. It's a prison. Why am I here? I'm a prisoner."

Dunham and Weinberg (1960:4-5) note:

> The mental patient is often a highly sensitive person who desires safe, quiet and private surroundings. In the mental hospital this sensitive person is thrown into a situation where his every act and utterance becomes the public property of strangers--his fellow patients and the hospital employees. Dressing, eating, toileting, sleeping, talking are done constantly under the watchful eyes of persons charged with his care. With this constant public invasion of what for normal people constitutes much of their privacy, these highly sensitive and emotional persons must come to terms. Thus, the type of adjustment demanded from mental patients is often of such a character as to cause a normal person to rebel.

William Buchan (quoted in Dain 1964:39), in a popular medical book published in 1769, said of asylums: "These institutions, as they are generally managed, are far more likely to make a wise man mad than to restore a madman to his senses." Some observers maintain that there has been little change since these words were written. Szasz (1970:126-128), notable opponent of institutional psychiatry, calls the mental hospital "harmful for the inmates" and, citing the 1789 work of John Reid, a British physician, describes it as a "manufactory of madness."[8] Scull (1977:77, 95-96) says that recent research in social psychiatry shows that such hospitals "are fundamentally antitherapeutic institutions having a detrimental impact on their inmate populations "due to irremediable flaws in the basic structure of such places."

However, it should be noted that some patients find a compatible environment in some mental hospitals, and more. Barton (1966:14) introduces a concept of "institutional neurosis":

> The term "neurosis" is used rather than "psychosis", since the syndrome itself does not interfere with the patient's ability to distinguish between reality and fantasy. . . . Institutional neurosis is a disease characterized by apathy, lack of initiative, loss of interest more marked in things and events not immediately personal or present, submissiveness . . . . These signs vary in severity from the mute stuperose patient . . . to the active cheerful patient who enjoys the facilities available . . . but shows no desire to leave the hospital [and] shows no interest in plans for a future outside the hospital.

In my interviews in Peru, some patients were unhappy at being incarcerated while others seemed to be quite content. Here are some positive extracts from the patient protocols:

> Patient Aguila: I like it because it's large. It's well ventilated. I like the care by the doctors and the nurses. Also the radio with its loudspeakers, which has made for a pleasant atmosphere. Then, as for the patients, there are a good number of them with whom I rub elbows in a friendly way. Since they have games, chess, checkers, and other parlor games, for those people who are in condition to play them it's something to do. They find comfort and distraction which benefits their spirits a great deal, improving some and making it possible for others to pass their time.
>
> Patient Chocano: This pavilion is a modern, comfortable one, well ventilated, with enough light and cleanliness. With enough comfort, it could be said. They even give us the luxury of having vegetable gardens. And it could be said that it looks like a crystal palace, with its modern dining room, even though it doesn't have a good chef. Well, what are we going to do! The patients live peacefully and they live well. They have come to get used to it. And some don't want to leave any more.
>
> Patient Ortiz: Pavilion 20 is elegant.
>
> Patient Peña: I like it here because it's very clean and has a lot of space. It is very large, very clean. I'm happy. I enjoy myself as much as anyone.
>
> Patient Armas: Pavilion 20 agrees with me because there are more patients, more people. I have a lot of companions, many friends. . . . Here there's plenty of glass in the windows.

Insane asylums are poor, coercive, and occasionally violent. Wing and Brown (1970:177-178) show the relationship between environmental poverty and a "clinical poverty syndrome." From a psychoanalytic point of view, the violent character of such institutions can be interpreted in terms of what Kris (1975:242) calls "retaliatory castration," that is, "the turning of a passive experience into an active one."[9] Taking a broader psychiatric perspective, Lion (1988:164) points out:

> There is no such diagnosis as "violent patient"; violence can be seen in manic-depressive illness, agitated depression, intermittent explosive

> disorders, alcoholism, or sexual paraphilia. The point to be made is that aggression is a symptom that cuts across many diagnostic entities. The clinician confronted with "a violent patient" needs to consider whether the violence is a manifestation of the subculture, an affective disease process, an incipient psychosis, a character disorder, a disorder of impulse control, an attention-deficit disorder, an organic mental disorder, or any of a variety of other illnesses that have complex behavioral characteristics.

To single out the mental hospital as a violent place in a society like that of the United States, or of Peru, is absurd because we live in violent habitats. Mechanic (1980:199) says:

> Violence is commonplace in our society. Most persons who engage in violent, destructive, or other harmful behaviors are not mentally ill unless the behaviors are defined as criteria for judging illness, which would be tautological. All of us pose some risks to others--by the way we live, the way we drive, the extent to which we take precautions to avoid accidents, and so on. Psychiatrists' conceptions of danger include a tendency toward personal violence, such as attacks on persons or property. A businessperson who sells defective products or a manufacturer who fails to report a known safety defect in a product may do far more harm to others than a mentally ill person but would not usually be included within the psychiatric conception.

Martini P. (1983:33) says: "The psychiatric hospital is intrinsically violent, since its official purposes consist of forcibly adapting inmates to the rules of the institution." Cooper (1967:14) says that, "in fact, violence in psychiatry is pre-eminently the violence *of* psychiatry." And, speaking of the incarcerative aspect, Levinson and Gallagher (1964) ask if, even with contemporary reforms, it would be possible to avoid deleterious effects on patients:

> One question is worth noting . . .: How far can mental hospitals go in minimizing the incarcerative aspect of patienthood? As hospitals now function, this is usually a prominent aspect, and it undermines the more constructive functions. For the great majority of patients, hospitalization could be much more an opportunity than a legal sentence, and the hospital more a therapeutic-educative ally than an oppressive machine. Attempts to encourage voluntary admission by patients, to develop the open hospital, and to regard patients as active

> participants in the therapeutic enterprise, are steps in this direction. How far these changes can go is indeed a moot question.

The asylum's coercion, nevertheless, does not always have to be objective and obvious; rather, it can be subjective and subtle. Foucault (246-247) notes that, with the beginning of so-called "moral treatment", in place of the brutality of earlier madhouses, "The obscure guilt that once linked transgression and unreason is thus shifted; the madman, as a human being originally endowed with reason, is no longer guilty of being mad; but the madman, as a madman, and in the interior of that disease of which he is no longer guilty, must feel morally responsible for everything within him that may disturb morality and society, and must hold no one but himself responsible for the punishment he receives." Thus, while the asylum ceased punishing the mad person's guilt, "it did more, it organized that guilt." Thus, also, according to Goffman (1962:306, 206), the hospital "outmaneuvers the patient", since "everything a patient is caused to do can be described as a part of his treatment or of custodial management; everything a patient does on his own can be defined as symptomatic of his disorder or of his convalescence." Or, as Scull (1979:202) observes, a great contradiction arises:

> [T]he creation of . . . expensive specialized institutions in the first place had drawn its legitimacy from the constantly reiterated contention that lunatics were sick and/or not responsible for their own actions. Yet, if these vast asylums were to operate at all, patients had to be made to conform to the rules of the institutions, and this could only be done by utilizing the ordinary system of rewards and punishments to elicit the desired behavior. But the resort to positive and negative sanctions was a tacit concession that it made some sort of sense to hold the lunatic responsible for his actions, and that by doing so his behaviour could be manipulated. In practice, then, the definition of actions as symptoms could not be maintained if the institution was to continue to function, and could scarcely be discarded if asylum doctors were to continue to maintain the fiction that their work was esentially medical in character.

Elsewhere, Scull (1991:154) adds to this:

> To see in all this only the benevolent face of moral treatment--its break with the crude coercion of the past--is to ignore the latent

Elsewhere, Scull (1991:154) adds to this:

> To see in all this only the benevolent face of moral treatment--its break with the crude coercion of the past--is to ignore the latent power of these techniques as a mechanism for enforcing conformity. The pervasive authority of the alienist . . . constituted an extraordinary powerful new form of "moral machinery", a superior mode of *managing* patients. The use of space in the form of the ward system to constitute and make salient moral boundaries, and the creation of an intimate tie between the patient's position in this classificatory system and his behavior, enabled alienists to use every aspect of the environment as "a more powerful lever in acting upon the intractable." It was precisely the hidden strengths of moral treatment as a mechamism for the management and regulation of conduct and the production of docile bodies which made possible the abandonment of the brutal and harsh methods of management which had previously been inextricably connected with the concentration of large numbers of lunatics in an institutional environment. And in placing far more effective and through-going means of control in the hands of the custodians, while simultaneously removing the necessity for the asylum's crudest features, the reality of that imprisonment and control simultaneously became far more difficult to perceive.

Goffman (1962:385) concludes: "The point is not that the hospital is a hateful place for patients but that for the patient to express hatred of it is to give evidence that his place in it is justified and that he is not yet ready to leave it." Szasz (1970:278) says: "The feared violence of the madman is . . . best understood as largely the projection, onto the victim, of the actual violence of his persecutor." As Cooper (1967:97, 103) puts it, mental hospital personnel defend themselves against their own madness by confronting it in their patients. At the same time, violence engenders violence; and if the asylum uses force, although this may be hidden and subtle rather than naked and brutal in our times, the popular image of an insane person is a violent one. In terms which have contemporary relevance, Tomes (1984:188-189, 239) speaks of a "therapeutic persuasion" held by North American psychiatric personnel of the nineteenth century which was often not shared by the patients, the nature of whose disturbance "made them unable or unwilling to accept the premises of asylum treatment," so that "for the patient determined to defy the hospital's authorities, physical violence was another dramatic form of resistance." Thus, the "security" measures imposed by the asylum, as Greenblatt (1955:45) points out in regard to the traditional institution, "were essentially self-defeating, since they tended to promote a feeling of restriction and repression, of fear and punitiveness. . . . [They] failed to reduce the disturbed behavior . . [or] prevent escape. The patient proved equal to the challenge of turning heavy furniture to diabolical ends . . . [and] fires frequently broke out in remote corners of the corridors, and even in seclusion rooms in which patients had been locked."

Despite the violence characteristic of the public image of the "lunatic," most mental patients are not violent.[10] Mechanic (1980:200) states:

> Contrary to popular conceptions, studies suggest that in the aggregate mental patients are no more dangerous than others or if they are, the differences are very small allowing little success in prediction. The public's more clear-cut perception results in part from the prominence given by the news media to the former-mental-patient status of those who commit serious crimes. Such associations reinforce a perceived link that is at odds with statistical reality. . . . The validity of clinical conceptions of danger and violence has not been established, and there is every reason to believe that violence is specific to situation and context and not simply an attribute of a person.

In his study of insanity in California during the last decades of the last century and the first decades of the present one, with data from commitment examiners' reports for admissions to a San Francisco hospital, Fox (1978:142-143, 152) notes that only ten per cent of the examined persons exhibited "violence," and adds that "more than one-third of the 'violent' behavior contained in the category of threats was directed against official personnel: policemen, doctors, nurses, and others. Such violence may in some cases have been less a symptom of disability than a response to detention." The evidence leads this author to conclude:

> If the individuals committed for insanity by the San Francisco Superior Court posed a threat, it was ordinarily not a threat to other persons, property, or themselves, but to articulated moral norms, to the culture's underlying sense of "reality," or to the peace and tranquility of their relatives, neighbors, or public officials.

Mental hospital personnel themselves, appropriately or

inappropriately, often contribute to patient violence, when it occurs.[11] Soloff (1983:249-250) points out that staff conduct in relation to the patient makes "a major impact on the violence of his behavior." If the staff attitude, derived possibly "from projection of their own anger at the potentially combative patient," is "dominated by fear and anger," such "countertransference reactions may lead to defensive denial on the part of the clinician or, conversely, a violent overreaction. A sustained state of anxiety and fear among staff is intolerable and invariably leads to a forced resolution. The 'dangerous patient' may actually be encouraged to 'act out' his potential, justifying staff retaliation and discharge of tension into action."

The Peruvian hospital is no exception. All the categories of personnel related tales of patient assaultiveness. We may begin with some of the doctors, of whom only six of the twelve interviewed told me that they had never experienced attacks:

> Dr. Alba: I was attacked only once in five years here. It was light. A woman tried to choke me with my tie. It happened because I didn't think it was important and I treated it as a joke. It was in Pavilion [n]. She began to straighten my tie and then she choked me. I pushed her away and that was all.

> Dr. Bueno: I've never worried about physical danger, though patients have tried to attack me on several occasions. Once, when I was giving electroshock treatments, I remember one patient quite well. Every time I arrived in Pavilion [n], he was waiting for me like a wild animal, but I always had that fierce man called to the treatment room. After more than fifteen applications, one morning the patient embraced me in one of the corridors, but an employee always followed me as a guard. The patient embraced me in order to tell me that he was very grateful because thanks to the treatments I had given him he had improved. Not just that one but many patients who had behaved poorly with me have thanked me. I had to excuse them because it's a matter of the illness.
>
> On another occasion, in one of the rooms--I was giving treatments in private houses--we found an iron bar for some assault. I don't know if it was for me or some other doctor, but I have never gone into rooms for treatment without first looking for something under the mattress of every patient. That was my habit and it was the job of the employee who always watched the disturbed patients.

> Dr. Espinoza: One never knows when a patient will have an

aggressive impulse. One takes care. . . . Once there was an attempt by a patient. He thought I was taking the side of two other patients who were complaining about him. Another attempt was by another patient. It was mistaken identity. He thought I was Dr. Bueno.

Dr. Herrera: On two occasions, before antipsychotic drugs were in use, two patients maneuvered aggressively around me, without consequences, and they were stopped without other measures than deepening the interpersonal relations both times.

While some nurses also told me that they had never experienced attacks on their persons, others mentioned assaultive incidents:

Nurse Arruga: I've worked most of my professional life among men, but once when I was a student I was attacked in a pavilion for women. She tried to choke me and I protected myself. The attendant came, but by that time I'd managed to pacify the woman.

Nurse Chivas: Injuries are quite frequent. One is like an authority here and they can take one for one of their enemies. I've seen a series of things, many accidents on the personnel's part. In Pavilion [n] you'll see a man whose ear is bitten off. One has to be very careful and know the patients well. The same patient attacked me. He bit my arm. Everybody has been hurt. They've hurt me about ten times. The last time was three months ago in Pavilion [n]. It was an assault, a punch, because I was careless. What we do is this: we try to evade it until we can call the resident physician or another person. Then on the next day we inform the pavilion doctor.

Nurse Godoy: One forgets what can happen to one. We aren't continually worried about it. Sure, inside a men's pavilion a person has to be more careful, but this is more when she doesn't know the patients. They never have attacked me. I haven't had the bad luck, and still I've worked in a men's pavilion. There are signs when they're disturbed. Then we give them injections. That's why we have attendants, to be alert for what can happen. They always hold a patient who is beginning to be assaultive. One woman here gets violent when she has crises; she even grabs bricks and throws them. Everybody runs away from her, but when I get near her she never does me any harm.

Nurse Hurtado: Of course, one has to walk around carefully. A mental patient can have different reactions at different times. We keep on the alert. I'm only worried when I'm on this service. In ten years of managing mental patients I was slapped on the face once. It wasn't a man but a woman. My rule is that I try not to let myself be grabbed and I try to get free, in any way I can, from a disturbed patient, or to prevent it with immediate assistance from the attendants.

More attendants talked about assaults, doubtlessly because they are more frequently in contact with patients than other categories of personnel:

Attendant Estrada: I don't worry about the danger. If a person comes to work here, he does it willingly. If bad luck comes, then it comes, but during seven years here nothing's happened to me. Of course I've been threatened, but they've never hit me because it's always been possible for me to prevent them. Once in Pavilion [n] a patient hit me and I fell on the floor. But we can't hit them. That's forbidden. We can hold them. Here, when the nurse was trying to give a patient an injection, and we had to hold him, he gave me a punch on my mouth. I had a bloody nose.

Attendant García: The day before yesterday, while I was taking a patient back to his bed, another patient kicked me. One has to be careful.

Attendant Jiménez: Yes, I've been attacked around six or seven times. Just recently it happened to me. I was cleaning in dormitory six and a patient came to my side. He wanted to take the mop handle to hit me with it. A week ago I was in the insulin treatment room and suddenly a patient became disturbed. He began to shout a lot of insulting things to me. He started to get near me, hitting out and throwing things. The only thing I could do was to try to pacify him, but when I saw that he was not settling down, I told the nurse. Ten days before that I was also attacked.

Attendant León: They still haven't hurt me, but they've done it to others. When my brother was working in Pavilion [n], a patient almost killed him. He was working in the wardrobe and he had a patient to help him, one who had the habit of attacking employees. My brother was busy and careless. The patient jumped on him from above. He had to go to the doctor for six months. He got well, but he doesn't work here any more.

Attendant Meza: The last time I was attacked was six months ago. A patient got angry when I told him that it was forbidden for him to be in the dispensary. That's when he attacked me. He hit me once and I managed to avoid anything more. That's all that happened.

Attendant Nores: They've attacked me around three times. The last one was three years ago. I was serving lunch and I told a young woman to eat. She grabbed my hair and threw me on the floor. I called the other attendants to come and help me. They came and helped me up. There are always slaps and kicks. When they bathe, some of them are afraid of the water, but there are always several employees and we can force them to do it.

Attendant Ortiz: One time a patient was in the therapy room, banging on the door. The nurse didn't notice that she was so disturbed. Another attendant opened the door and she jumped out. She settled on me because I was the closest. Fortunately the other attendants were there and grabbed her. We put her to bed. [She shows me a scar on her forehead and a broken fingernail.] That happened to me a month ago. It was the only time. Of course they are little things that always happen. They bother a person more with words. Sometimes they hit you when you are trying to separate them when they are fighting.

If violent incidents happen to the personnel, it seems that everyone in the hospital world recognizes that it is strictly prohibited to exercise violence upon the person of a patient, even though this occurs now and then. Two nurses specifically mentioned this possibility in their responses to my question on how a nurse can be discharged from his/her position in the hospital:

Nurse Arruga: A nurse can be discharged for a serious offense against the patients or against the institution. If one orders the employees to do something against the patients' health, or if one allows them to strike them. Also, if one leaves medicine or dangerous sharp things around where the patients can injure themselves, or if one leaves the service unattended.

Nurse Chivas: I've seen them fire nurses here. There are three kinds of punishment: One is for a light offense where they warn a person. Another is for a serious offense, like hitting a patient. If that is discovered the nurse is suspended. Third, if it's very serious, they fire him.

The attendants responded to the same question with more detail:

Atendant Alfaro: I saw a man fired just because they found him playing cards. There could have been other offenses. They fired another man for fighting with a patient. He knocked the patient's teeth out. When the nurse saw him doing that he told him he had been behaving bad with the patients. It wasn't the first time. He'd had two or three offenses. They threw him out.

Attendant Chacón: Smoking is not allowed, nor is abusing the patients. Sometimes attendants are let go because they played cards during working hours, or because they were absent from the service. They excuse a person for absence for one or two days, but after the third day they fire him. Also for patient escapes, for insubordination, or for disrespect to the bosses [i.e., nurses].

Atttendant García: One can be discharged for being absent for three days, or for something serious one has committed during work, for disrespect, or for hitting someone. They punish an attendant by suspending him for one or two weeks, but if it's really serious they fire him. There was a man who worked here for twenty-five years. He had sexual relations with a woman patient. They threw him out for raping the patient. He had no recourse. Fighting with the nurses or doctors is a serious thing, but it never happens.

Attendant Hoyos: For not being obedient sometimes, that is, not obeying an order from the nurse, or also for unfairly maltreating a patient. For missing work or when attendants fight with each other. One can return by making a complaint, appearing at the union for hospital workers. It depends on the case. Sometimes the administration itself arranges things.

Atendant Ibáñez: They can fire an attendant for hitting a patient, for an absence of two or three days or for contradicting a nurse. In other pavilions I've seen cases, but never here. Another worker in Pavilion [n] hit a patient who had kicked him. The patient, all bloody, came to the nurse to complain. The nurse went to the superintendant's and the attendant was fired immediately, exactly because an attendant has no right to strike a patient. It's better to go away in order to avoid a misfortune. There's no reason to hit somebody.

Atendant Jiménez: For example, an attendant can be fired from the job for disobeying a superior's orders or not following them, and when an attendant hits a patient or when he behaves badly with a superior or offends him. About three months ago they fired an attendant because he hit a nurse, and he'd also maltreated the patients. He hit the nurse because he came to work drunk. The nurse told him he ought not to behave himself the way he was behaving, and the two of them had an exchange of words. That was the reason why they did what they did to the employee.

Atendant Llona: They can fire a person when he's absent a lot or when there's some kind of disorder on the service. Or when he's not on time. Also when he maltreats some patient. Or when, for some reason, he wants to take something from the hospital, in secret, without asking the nurse or somebody else in charge of the service.

Attendant Nores: One has to commit some serious offense. It would be for stealing or showing disrespect for a superior. I remember a case that was for theft. Almost all the cases are like that, or because the attendants were fighting among themselves or with the boss. Fighting between attendants and patients would have to be on the men's side.

Clearly, there exists a structural violence in the mental hospital which can be conceived as prior to the violent behavior of patients, in the senses of the locking up of patients, their subjection to the rules of the institution, the use of restraints, the practice of seclusion, enforced dependence on hospital authorities, the use of trickery, the system of rewards and punishments,[12] and, even at times, the recourse to force itself in compelling patients to obey. Goffman (1962:263, note 124) says: "Use of physical force by staff in mental hospitals for purposes presented as legitimate is a basic feature of patient life; some of its forms, such as forced feeding, prevention of suicide, or protecting one patient from another's attack, are not easily criticized," but note the author's use of qualifiers like "presented as legitimate" and "not easily criticized." It is the opinion of Szasz (1970:278) that "the feared violence of the madman is . . . best understood as largely the projection, onto the victim, of the actual violence of his persecutor."; nevertheless, Goffman (1962:368) points out, "a patient . . . may well feel he must fight and hate his keepers if any sense is to be made of the hardship he is undergoing." Martini P. (1983:43-44) describes the former structural location of those personnel of the Italian asylum, called "nurses," who appear more to resemble Peruvian attendants:

> On the lowest level of the institutional power pyramid the nurses were located. They had the riskiest role, at the same time the most unpopular one; They had to apply and force compliance with institutional norms in all aspects by direct contact with the patient. As may be expected, the relationship took on violent characteristics when the patient refused to obey the doctor's orders--the taking of medications, work rules, transfer to another hospital unit, and so on--. In every way, the relationship between the nurse and the patient was inevitably violent, since all the rights of the inmate were systematically denied and the nurses often discharged on the latter the frustration derived from poorly paid labor, with no prestige, lacking in autonomy, and potentially dangerous.

I asked the nurses and attendants a series of three questions about the use of force: "How do you get a patient up who doesn't want to get up?," "How do you get a patient to eat who doesn't want to eat?," and "Should force be used on patients?" (Unfortunately I did not ask these of the doctors.) There is no need to include all the responses here, but the following are representative:

> Nurse Arruga: He is just gotten up. It depends. Some are violent and then you need help from the attendants. With some, you just speak in an authoritative voice.
>
> You can suggest it [eating] to some of them. The negativists always try to fool you. So then you have to warn them that we're going to use the "*sonda*" [catheter or feeding tube].
>
> In general, a nurse ought not to use force, but in the event of an assault I have to defend myself and subdue the patient. That's not maltreating him but defending oneself.

> Nurse Bustos: We have to persuade them, talk to them.
>
> You have to make friends with them, gain their confidence and explain things to them.
>
> Really, a nurse shouldn't use force. We try to persuade them any way we can.

> Nurse Cruz: I tell the patient to get up two or three times, and he obeys. It's all a matter of not insisting.
>
> In the case of food, first I talk to him and I persuade him that food is necessary, that if he doesn't eat it will hurt him.

We can't hit them, but, sure, we can grab them. You can't hit them.

Nurse Chivas, only to the third question: Yes. Here they teach us in the nursing school about a series of holds, like wrestlers. Otherwise we'd be lost. So we can do something like that, until help comes. If we didn't have that skill, we could be hurt.

Nurse Esquivel, only to the third question: If it's necessary, of course, to subdue them. Once I broke my ribs grabbing a patient.

Attendant Alfaro: It depends on conditions, because there are attendants who treat patients as patients treat them. If they don't want to get up, the attendant goes to call the doctor. If they get up assaultive, the attendant has to grab them. If the patient is sick, he's left alone, but if he's not sick he is forced to get up. We have to serve him food. We grab him by the arm and tell him that the doctor has ordered it. That's where the trouble starts.

We have to feed him. The attendant has to take the spoon and open the patient's mouth. The nurse puts in a gadget to feed him, if necessary. It's called the *sonda*. The attendant looks on.

Yes, of course, one has to use force, and one has to do that a lot because if an employee is weak the patient hits him. If a patient attacks me, I have to grab him. There are sleeves with which a patient's arms are tied behind his back. We use them very seldom here, but a lot in Pavilion [n]. They're quite wild there.

Attendant Costa: If he doesn't get up, I tell him to. You can't get him up against his will. Sometimes the doctor says he should be gotten up and then, with two or three attendants, we make him.

If he doesn't eat, it's fed to him with a spoon and opening his mouth. The patient usually doesn't resist and then we urge him to eat.

Yes, sometimes force is used.

Attendant Chacón: If the patient is in that mood, he has to be gotten up anyway. One has to make him obey. One calls all the employees to help carry him.

With food, one takes a spoon and insists on feeding him. If he pushes the attendant's arm away, one has to call another employee to hold him.

It's necessary to use force when a patient is disturbed, when he doesn't want to take a bath, because sometimes they don't obey.

Attendant Estrada: If he doesn't want to get up, sure, he's gotten up. It depends on the nurse's orders. We take him and put him in the patio.

If he's not eating, we feed him through a *sonda*. You can't give him dry food, so we give him a beaten egg with milk or syrup.

Force can't be used on him.

Attendant García: When he doesn't get up, you have to dress him, wash him, and feed him. You take his arm and pull him.

When he doesn't want to eat one tells the nurse and he's the one who puts the tube up his nose.

If the patient is aggressive, one calls the nurse. Then it's necessary to use force to give him injections to calm him down.

Attendant Hoyos: It's necessary for them to get up. You have to do it in the best way. Even if it's by fooling them, you have to do it. You tell them, "I'm going to give you something," or "The doctor is calling you."

If he doesn't eat, one sits down beside him and feeds him with a spoon. If he pushes one's hand away, then it's necessary to use force.

Sometimes it's necessary to use force, for example, when he doesn't want to come when he's called.

Attendant Llona: The attendant gets him up by insisting that he get up, and if he doesn't want to, two of us attendants take him by the arm and dress him or make him dress himself.

If he doesn't eat he's fed by spoon. Today V_____ sat in front of his food for a long time without eating. I told him to eat and he said he had no appetite. So I took the spoon and fed him until he finished his lunch. My station was in the patio, that is, watching the patients there. The attendant who has that job has to stay with them, help serve lunch, and watch them to see that they eat.

Yes, force has to be used in cases when a patient is disturbed. It's necessary to prevent them from a disaster. It's necessary to hold them.

Attendant Nores: If they won't get up, you have to oblige them to. They can attack, but when they see you coming in a group of three they back down.

It's necessary to force her to eat with a spoon by several of us holding her.

Force must be used at the time they start something. If they drop on the floor or if they refuse an order, then we have to use force.

V

It should be emphasized that criticism of the asylum is not based on the presumed bad intentions or twisted motives of the personnel who, it would seem, try to do their jobs, give treatment or custodial care to their patients, and promote the good of the hospital world. Rather, the contradiction exists in the structure of the institution; it is, as was pointed out at the beginning of this Chapter, a structural ambivalence. As psychiatric specialists have slowly come to an awareness of this feature of their enterprise they had not been conscious of earlier, the practice of psychiatry has changed. M. Jones (1953:36), who is to be credited with the popularization of the concept, "therapeutic community," notes that "the main problem confronting us . . . is how to clarify our different staff roles, and, having done so, how to work as harmoniously as possible as an integrated whole. But along with this, at every stage, is the imperative necessity to convey to the patients an awareness of this structure so that it is as well known to them as to ourselves."

Nothing that has been said so far indicates that the mental hospital should be abolished, in spite of the severe criticism it has received. Kubie (1975:389-390) defends hospital psychiatry by pointing out that critics who attack mental hospitals in support of human rights "fail to realize that the very essence of psychological illness is the impairment or actual loss of psychological freedom"; that the elimination of mental hospitals is "short-sighted and mercenary . . . because [other critics] erroneously think it would save the taxpayer's money"; and that still other critics focus on what hospitals "do not do, without realizing that it is the lack of adequate funding that makes it impossible for them to have adequate staffs and adequate facilities . . . but these attacks contribute to the starvation rations on which hospitals are required to live and then are criticized for what they cannot supply." Grob (1983:318-319) says:

> The one-sided notion that all mental hospital care was no more than abuse of patients . . . precluded consideration of some probable consequences of closing down all mental hospitals. . . . With all of its shortcomings, [the mental hospital] was among the few institutions that provided some minimal basic care for persons whose mental and physical condition--whatever the origins of this condition--rendered

> them dependent upon others for their very survival. This basic fact alone--to say nothing about those individuals who benefitted from their confinement and were able to return to the community--should have tempered the unyielding attack on the legitimacy of mental hospital care. To patients the choice was not between mental hospital forms of care and other alternatives; the choice at the time was between institutional care or no care at all.

Thus, as in other parts of the world where the historical trend of the growth of mental hospitals has been reversed (see Martini P. 1983, Scull 1977, Talbott 1978), Peruvian psychiatric care has been decentralized and diffused. Mariátegui (1988:70) observes:

> The time of large psychiatric hospitals with long-term stays has definitely approached its end; the system of small establishments and specialized departments in general hospitals, articulated with a network of peripheral centers, allows for a developing management of illness in intimate contact with the community. . . . In this way we are overcoming the traditional objectives of the organization of psychiatric care based on large, specialized establishments, emphasizing the conception of the promotion of Mental Health, and giving priority to prevention, early treatment, rehabilitation, and reintegration into the community.

Chamberlin (1978:7) speaks of the desirability of "true asylums, places to which people can retreat to deal with the pain of their existence." Estroff (1981:254) believes "that clients, and all of us, still need a place to rest or to be crazy if necessary." M. Jones (1968:137) offers this defense of the asylum:

> The old term "asylum", dissociated from the stigma applied by a society fearful of mental illness, is in fact . . . appropriate. People who are unable to cope with the stress of ordinary life should be allowed to find asylum of a temporary kind, where with understanding, support, and psychotherapeutic treatment they may be rehabilitated back to the world outside. For patients who cannot ever expect to cope in the outside world with a society as at present constituted, or for patients who are liable to have a protracted stay in hospital, the whole concept of the hospital should be changed to something more akin to a village settlement. In such a setting, the rehabilitation goal would be to afford the individual the optimal role compatible with his disability, personality, and assets. . . . The

> examination of the role of the patient under these projected conditions would almost certainly lead to the disappearance of the term "patient" and also of the present concept of the role relationship between patient, psychiatrist, nurse, and so on.

Scull (1979:262), who has contributed much to current discussion critical of the asylum, points out:

> But realism about the awfulness of asylum existence ought not to prompt us to opt for a blind faith in the virtues of its presumed antithesis. One can--indeed, I think must--be deeply sceptical about claims made on the mental hospital's behalf: yet one must not fall prey to equally groundless fantasies and illusions about the available alternatives.

The alternative of deinstitutionalization, or "decarceration" (see Scull 1977), and the setting up of "community mental health centers" was in the 1960's and 1970's thought to be a solution to asylumdom. Morrissey, Goldman, and Klerman (1980:2-3) describe the process:

> These dual objectives were made plausible by changes in psychosocial treatment approaches, by the discovery and widespread use of psychotropic drugs, and by the growing availability of federally financed community mental health centers, of nursing homes, and of general hospital-based psychiatric services. . . . Already there are unmistakable signs that the "bold new approach" embodied in this reform has created new problems and left many old ones unsolved. Thousands of "deinstitutionalized" patients have been returned to communities only to encounter hostility and rejection by citizens and the new community centers alike. Many severely and chronically disabled patients have been "dumped" in the rooming houses and decaying hotels of innercity areas while other tends of thousands have been "reinstitutionalized" in nursing homes and chronic care facilities. Still others who remained in state hospitals have suffered and even died because the resources essential to maintain adequate care have been shifted to community-based agencies.

Kraft (1981:364) says:

> All other things being equal, it may be better for a patient to live in the community. But often, all other things are not equal. Patients discharged from mental hospitals have found themselves in inadequate

> single-room occupancy dwellings, poorly managed proprietary care homes, hotels, and, too often, jails. The quest for moving patients out of hospitals has led to poorly conceived and inadequate alternative arrangements. Every patient is *not* better off outside the hospital.

And Estroff (1981:253-254) comments:

> De-institutionalization has, for the most part, been simplistically effected through movement away from the architectural embrace of hospitals. But institutions, of course, are complex, extending beyond walls to the articulation of traditions and values at a societal level. In this sense, the institutions of chronic mental illness have been little affected by the escape from institutional buildings. The roles, expectations, steoeotypes, and responses that accompany being a back-ward patient or a long-term community outpatient have changed little. It is as if we thought what was noxious to patients was somehow present in the actual walls of hospitals.

Thus, the setting up of community-centers in the disintegrating cores of urban areas in North America, without secure financing or staffs that quite understand their purposes, is not a rational, constructive, or positive response to the continued existence of madness. The reform movement which seemed so full of hope, with much promise of social and cultural construction, is shown in retrospect to have been guided by legislators who were more appalled by rising asylum costs than by terrible asylum conditions, as revealed by very vocal critics who provided a good rationale for cutting those costs and dumping masses of former mental patients into spaces inhabited by minority populations, victims of structural violence themselves, who could not or would not protest, or whose protests were not heard by the white majority. As Luske (1990:10) observes:

> The chief beneficiaries of the community psychiatric movement have been psychiatric professionals and nursing home interests. The former group saw in this movement a way to challenge medical psychiatry's virtual monopoly over psychiatric policy, as well as the opportunity for increased influence on its direction. They failed in their first objective, but succeeded in obtaining more lucrative and influential jobs as middle managers and clinicians within the burgeoning psychiatric bureaucracies. And the nursing home industry as a whole has turned a tidy profit from the government transfers, i.e., taxes, from which state medical insurance pays for treatment in a

community.

Sharkey (1994:177) sarcastically comments:

> By the 1980s, with private health-insurance money flooding into the high end of the mental-health and addiction treatment field, the record of deinstitutionalization was abundantly clear. In a 1981 editorial, *The New York Times* called the policy "a cruel embarassment, a reform gone terribly wrong." The evidence of that failure was all around. "Not since the 1820s have so many mentally ill individuals lived untreated in public shelters, on the streets and in jails," said a report commissioned in 1990 by the Public Citizen Health Research Group and the National Alliance for the Mentally Ill. The report declared that the largest "de facto mental hospital in the U.S. is the Los Angeles County jail, where there are 3,600 inmates who are seriously mentally ill on an average day," seven hundred more than were in the nation's largest mental hospital. Charging that psychiatry had abandoned the severely mentally ill for lucrative private practices or the lure of investor-owned hospitals, the report concluded that there had been a "near total breakdown in public psychiatric services in the United States."

Constructive change comes hard. Kiesler and Sibulkin (1987:205) point out the political-economic framework in which innovation must function:

> Thoroughly overhauling our mental health policy would not be a simple matter, however badly needed. The political constraints against massive policy change are enormous, even if one can demonstrate that the total cost would not be increased. There is ordinarily considerable resistance to any organizational change, a principle to which the U.S. Congress and state legislatures are no exception. The vested interest in mental health policy include various professional organizations, powerful drug companies, and unions of workers in institutional settings. These groups are politically powerful and have resisted change in the past. The AMA [American Medical Association], for example, has opposed every major piece of social legislation affecting health delivery in the last 50 years, including Social Security, Medicaid, and Medicare.

In Latin America, poverty is the major problem. Even if there were no political-economic constraints on how health budgets are to be used,

Peru and its neighbors, plagued with external debt and desperate search for income sources, must spend less and less on health care and other public welfare measures which should be human rights everywhere. Alarcón (1990:644) comments:

> The number of psychiatric beds on the Latin American sub-continent has not increased in the last decade, or if it has done so the increment has been extremely modest. Similarly, there has been no growth in the number of psychiatric hospitals or hospitalization services, outpatient departments, or sources of mental health referral. Rather, the impression exists that the number of these facilities has diminished in relation to population increase and psychiatric morbidity. To speak of community centers for mental health, rehabilitation centers, day hospitals, protected workshops. occupational therapy centers, or similar facilities, only means listing a collection of pleasant hopes or ideal resources. The situation is not improving if we include the provision of medications or psychopharmaceutical agents in the list of material resources: either they are not supplied in an adequate quantity because of distribution problems, or they are not within the reach of majorities because of their high cost, or, simply, they are not produced or imported suficiently to meet the demand.

In some parts of Latin America, a parallel process of deinstitutionalization is taking place. González Uzcátegui (1991:159) comments:

> In some locations the choice has been to favor the progressive depopulation of psychiatric hospitals, restricting admissions and opting for the placement of patients in shelters, foster homes, self-governing collectives, and other modes of care in the community. In other places the intention has been to empty the asylums without offering a sufficient number of alternatives, and the results have been catastrophic for the welfare of patients who have been "reintegrated into the community." Elsewhere, alternatives to hospitalization only mean the removal to another facility, frequently more uncomfortable for the patient, removed from the doctrines and practice of asylum treatment.

Within these realities, asylums are still needed and will continue to be. Castel, Castel, and Lovell (1982:105) note in regard to the situation in North America: "Quantitatively, the state hospitals are still the most important resource for inpatient care of mental illness: in 1974 two-thirds of the beds available for psychiatric patients were in state mental hospitals. State hospitals also lead in the number of cases treated, accounting for more than a third of all cases treated in hospital. The state hospitals employ more than half of all mental health workers and 61 percent of the hospital staff, and they consume more than a third of the mental health budget and more than half the hospital budget."

It is clear, therefore, despite all the problems and constraints which have been outlined, that consultation anthropology in the sense of the transmission of information back to hospital staff by an ethnographic observer (see Stein 1993) can be useful, if it can reveal something of the structural ambivalence which appears to lie in the nature of such institutions, as well as in the nature of their political and economic contexts, to the persons who operate them. Freud's goal, as stated in his maxim, "Where id was, there ego shall be," can be applied to institutions and states as well as it can be to individuals. It is utopian, surely, but the mere fact that we never can learn all there is to know about ourselves should not prevent us *ever* from the continuing process of learning a little more.

Notes

1. Goffman's sociological study is excellent, without question. However, I believe that its publication assisted the demise of mental hospital "ethnographies." There was little more to be said about the tragic conditions in large public hospitals after he had spoken. At the same time, beyond the refocusing of sociological attention, psychiatric reaction developed: K. Jones (1982:221) observes: "Many psychiatrists ceased to read sociology after the publication of Goffman's *Asylums* because it seemed that sociology was off on some kind of ego-trip which was deeply antithetical to their own professional experience." We may well wonder what favors Goffman was conferring on whom. Grob (1994:264) says: "Goffman's own portrait of mental institutions was devastating; he described the ways in which a humiliating institutionalization stripped individuals of their self-identity and esteem and induced deviant responses. . . . *Asylums* was the product of a gifted and perceptive observer. Its literary and intellectual qualities were striking, and often overshadowed the methodological difficulties inherent in relying solely on personal observations. . . . Goffman's commitment to individual autonomy and a kind of eccentricity ensured that he would be far removed from many public issues. Nor did he offer any prescriptions for better and more effective ways of dealing with individuals designated as mental patients."

Goffman's work is not to be accepted uncritically. Sedgwick (1982:61-63) makes some useful observations: "Goffman's general assumption in *Asylums* is that there is no alternative to the way in which we treat mental patients in the public wards. . . . A 'functional explanation' is here presented as a means of avoiding questions of *policy towards inmates*, and of the moral responsibility both of society and of its official agents who administer the closed institution. . . . Erving Goffman, then, is not to be classed as a critical social theorist. His method consists in a precocious sensitivity toward those elements of social living which involve the face-to-face adjacency of persons. On all other aspects of the social process, that is to say, on any institution or happening that receives its meaning from outside this immediately shared space . . . he is virtually silent."

Mechanic (1980:129-130) comments: "Although Goffman made us aware of many aspects of total institutions that can be harmful to patients, we must recognize that total institutions can have good or deleterious effects depending on a variety of factors. Total institutions--hospitals, monasteries, schools--are organizations for changing people and their identities. If clients share the goals and aspirations of the organization, their experiences in it may be worthwhile and desirable. If clients are involuntarily admitted and reject the identity the institution assigns them, residence in such an organization may be extremely stressful and lead to profound disabilities in functioning. . . . Our attention should focus not on whether a hospital fits the model of a total institution but rather on specifying those aspects of such institutions that affect their performance."

2. It would seem that almost from the time that mental hospitals were first constructed critical evaluations of their performance also appeared. For the social history of psychiatry and psychiatric hospitals in Britain and the United States, see Grob (1966, 1973, 1979, 1983, 1991, 1994), McGovern (1985), Scull (1979, 1981), and Tomes (1984).

3. Carlos Alberto Seguin (*in* Alarcón 1990:591) denies that Valdizán was a psychiatrist but says that he "was a magnificent physician and an exceptional man; more than a psychiatric technician, he was a psychiatric humanist." It seems to me, however, that during those early days of this century psychiatrists were self-made.

4. I have reported, in Chapter 1, on the responses of the doctors to this question combined with another on the goals of the hospital, and so there is no need to include all of them here.

5. Peru has two systems of social security, one for *obreros*, blue-collar workers, and another for *empleados*, white-collar workers. It is a sad commentary on economic conditions in the country that these systems do not include, nor can they afford to include, the majority of Peruvian workers, i.e., they exclude peasants, farm laborers, casual laborers, and an informal sector which includes masses of apparent petty proprietors who are really marginalized

proletarians.

6. Although attendants are classified as laborers (*obreros*) for Social Security purposes, they refer to themselves as "employees" (*empleados*).

7. Stanton and Schwartz (1954:89) acknowledge such "supplies" needed by a mental hospital as "institutional needs" necessary for it "to achieve its purposes." Smith and Levinson (1957:3-4) say: "All human organizations for work are self-serving in many important respects. This is as true of organizations devoted to the healing arts as it is of frankly financial organizations. In all working organizations we find a complex blending of instrumental and maintenance functions. In the former we see the goal-directed, purposive functions of the organization--the general needs it was established to serve. In the latter set of functions we see that an organization exists to persist."

8. The mental hospital, of course, has no monopoly on the function of making people sick, or sicker than they are. In her study of medical and surgical services of a general hospital, Coser (1962:85) reproduces this statement by a patient: "I couldn't sleep all night. The lady next to me had a nightmare and was shrieking. Across the hall there was one who had gotten a needle and she yelled till the ceiling came down, I'm telling yah. So I walked out to have a smoke and there in the television room was the family of one who had died across the hall. They were crying and lamenting. I'll be glad to get home to get some rest. If I stay here longer, I'm going to get sick." Coser comments, "The joke that the hospital makes you sick or wears you out is a standard one. Through such standard jests, personal experiences are transformed into sentiments that can be shared by all."

9. Grob (1985:89) comments in connection with his reproduction of psychiatric correspondence regarding one hospital administration's discharge of attendants in 1928 for abuse of patients: "The threat of violence in mental hospitals was perennial. Some patients proved disruptive and threatened both themselves and others with physical harm. Some attendants used extreme force, sometimes without adequate justification."

10. Assaultive incidents in hospitals are not exclusive to psychiatric facilities but occur in emergency rooms, medical and surgical services, pediatrics, and other hospital departments. In their study of a university general hospital, Conn and Lion (1983:62) found that only 41 per cent of assaults "occurred within psychiatric units."

11. Snyder (1983:159), writing about a Maryland hospital, defends restraint: "[V]ery violent and combative wrestling and restraining may be unavoidable in the process of physically controlling an agitated patient. On some of our wards, primarily admission wards, physical restraint is almost a daily occurrence, and it is viewed by the staff as a necessary treatment proceedure for a patient during a disruptive and unstabilized point in his or her hospitalization. Patients, however, do not always view being restrained in like manner; in fact, restraint

may seem to them to be an instance of abuse and mistreatment. One need not be delusional to feel that way--the average person would probably agree that restraint is abusive."

12. See Spiegel's (1957:555-566) discussion of the processes of "role induction": coercion ("the manipulation of present and future punishments"), coaxing ("the manipulation of present and future rewards"), evaluating ("praising, blaming, shaming, approving and disapproving"), masking ("pretending, evading, censoring, distorting, lying, hoaxing, deceiving"), postponing, and role reversal--all of these techniques, some of them quite subtle, for changing behavior.

Chapter 4

Being a Mental Patient in Peru

What is it like to be a mental patient in Peru? How does one feel? What does one do? What problems does one have? What happens to one? What is one's vision of the hospital world? And what effect does the perspective of this sector constituting the overwhelming majority of the hospital population have on the therapeutic goals of the hospital? The purpose of this Chapter is to begin to frame a reply to these questions with data from my interviews with the patients of one pavilion of the Hospital Víctor Larco Herrera.

Before I proceed with the task I have outlined, some preliminary observations may be made with regard to more theoretical considerations. To begin, it is worth emphasizing that being a mental patient anywhere is fundamentally a *political* state. Because "insanity" is a social construction, and in view of the "conflicting goals and limited resources" of a society, persons with more power are to be found "managing" other persons; therefore, Romanucci-Ross (1983:280) states:

> In declaring mad persons to be "ill," psychiatry allows them to achieve patienthood and thereby to receive therapy, caring, and

> nurturance. But the label of mental "illness" carries with it a significant reduction in individual rights and responsibilities, and what began as a well-intentioned scientific and value-free advance also turned out to have important negative consequences. Even when all is circumspect in the diagnosis of insanity, the subsequent hospitalization and therapy--the entire process--is a *political* experience.

It is also useful to point out that both the structure that has been outlined as well as the deviance or the behavioral disorder of the individual produce feelings and needs in patients. Stanton and Schwartz (1954:169) note:

> To describe the role of the mental patient in the formal sense--as one complementary position in the doctor-nurse-patient triad within the broader mental hospital setting--is to run the risk of minimizing the vast amount of suffering the mental patient experiences, and to overlook the indefiniteness, complexity, and subtlety involved in "being a mental patient." It is hard to keep in mind what it means subjectively to be a mental patient; to be so fearful that each aspect of the environment represents a threat to one's existence; to experience the world as unreal and to see the "outside" as just a flimsy structure with no substance; to live with the feeling of restraint and being closed in, or suffocated, and to feel rebellion and resentment at this and be unable to express it in any effective way; to experience utter, desperate, and unrelieved loneliness, with no hope of change; to feel that in the entire universe there is no person that will ever understand one; to believe that one's actions have no effect and that one is not affected by the actions of others. To be a mental patient means to feel removed from the human race and to view oneself as not quite human; it means the inability to think or to trust one's thoughts; it means to be lacking in privacy and to be exposed to the view of strangers, and forced to associate with these strangers, when association with anyone is a thing to be dreaded and shunned.

We can also give some consideration to the patient's activities. What does he or she do within the hospital unit? How does he or she relate to other patients and to hospital personnel? In other words, we can examine the social role of the patient in the unit and in the hospital, not only as he or she enacts it but as he or she defines it. Furthermore, it is desirable to take into account what the patient adds to the life of the hospital world, for, as Parsons (1957:114) maintains, the patient does indeed contribute to the hospital process:

> There is a limiting type of somatic illness where the sick individual is simply an object being 'operated upon' by the therapeutic personnel. The only cooperation required of him then is to allow himself to be treated in this way; similarly with certain extreme psychoses. But corresponding to the fact that in mental illness the focus of disturbance is behavioral, is the fact that therapy is a process of social interaction. The positive role of the patient is an essential aspect of the process. His cooperation must be enlisted, he must be adequately motivated to "do his part" toward recovery. Therapy is cooperative "work."

However, the patient's vision includes more than feelings or social role: a patient also has combined with these an ideological perspective, formed before, during, and after his or her stay in the hospital, in which he or she explains the world he or she confronts in terms of his or her image of the hospital. Naboisek, et al. (1957:566-567) point out:

> Hospital image may be defined as a constellation of conscious and unconscious ideas and feelings about the hospital's purpose, ways of functioning, and personnel. . . . Deriving from many sources, internal and external, past and present, the ideas may be fixed, vague, contradictory, symbolic; the feelings, diffuse, hostile, repressed, etc.; or the opposites of any or all of these qualities may hold and in all combinations. . . . Even before actual contact with a mental hospital, people have conceptions about it, despite lack of even rudimentary understanding of mental illness, its causes, manifestations, treatment, and outcome. Popular stereotypes, however crude and sketchy, supply needed interpretations. Since cultural norms and directives are so often in conflict, much room is left for individual interpretation, so that which image is held is the reflection not only of cultural and social setting, but of individual personality factors as well.

In this context of the hospital's structure, the activities and feelings of patients, their definitions of their roles within the structure, and their images of the world which incorporates them, it may be said that they construct their own culture which, despite the ideological split between patients and personnel, influences hospital life. In this regard, Henry (1964:24-25) reports on his study of a mental hospital unit:

> An underlying assumption and therapeutic necessity in the operation

> of any healing institution is that it shall be controlled by the administration and administered benignly in the interest of the patients. When, however, we examine this ward, we discover that although in many respects the hospital did control the environment, the patients to a very considerable and important degree created their own *culture*. It is thus clear that in this respect the hospital was not "running" the patients; the patients were "running" the hospital. . . . [T]he employees appear to reinforce and to follow the norms of the patient culture. It appears likely that this was due to the fact that the employees shared the attitude of the patients. There was thus formed a kind of patient-personnel conspiracy to reproduce and reinforce on the ward the mirror image of the culture of the outer world.

All this does not contradict the possibility that in a unit there can exist disagreement, at times very strong, between patients and personnel. For example, Moos (1974:57-58) found in his study of 160 North American psychiatric units that there were significant differences between these sectors, enough to carry him to the conclusion that it was useful to conceptualize two distinct subcultures. Therefore, we may be facing the possibility that the two hospital population sectors can *unconsciously* hold beliefs, play roles, and construct images in regard to themselves and each other, which, as LeBar (1964:19) suggests, can animate and perpetuate "behavior not always in accord with therapeutic goals," which leads to the habitual acceptance of the patterns of unit life; in other words "institutionalism" (see Barton [1966] and Wing and Brown [1970]) can be as much a characteristic of the personnel as of the patients. Thus, Freidson's (1970a:60-61) critique of the medical profession has special relevance when it is applied to the psychiatric hospital: Freidson says that the goal of changing *individuals* instead of *social structures* is based on the supposition that "social pathologies connected with medical care, like illnesses connected with mankind, are 'caused' by the characteristics of the invididuals providing the care rather than by the environment in which the individuals provide care, and . . . that they are best treated by treating the individuals rather than the environment." However, it is possible for us to broaden our vision of the hospital world in such a way as to transform our individual approach to a collective approach.

I am going to deal with these themes here in the context of the observations and interviews I carried out in Pavilion 20 of the Lima Hospital, with emphasis on the patients. This pavilion, constructed in 1957 and therefore new within the Hospital, was a light, clean, and airy place, as "modern" as a psychiatric unit could be. It was equipped with games like chess, checkers, and cards; and there were always newspapers and magazines, not necessarily current ones, in circulation for those who liked to read. There was a physical education instructor in the Hospital who occasionally came to the pavilion to organize exercises or a football game. The pavilion was locked, although there was a breach in the wall which from time to time allowed a patient to leave without permission. At the time of the study, as was pointed out in Chapter 1, the pavilion contained around 70 internal male charity patients, eighty percent of whom were diagnosed as schizophrenics. With an informal question schedule I asked 27 of them,[1] ones who were able to speak with me, about their lives in the pavilion.

Before I explore what the patients told me about their Hospital lives, I would like to preface the report with some additional words about the content of their responses, particularly in view of the cautions I introduced in Chapter 2 in regard to my doubts about the utility of psychiatric patients" statements, that is, where the content might be contaminated by the nature of the subject's illness. It will be clear in some of the materials I will reproduce here that this is a relevant caution. At the same time, much of what the patients told me, I feel, can be used to construct of picture of what the life of the patient was like. Some of their responses, however, reveal some deformations, misunderstandings, and inappropriate statements that can be attributed to illness, but there are many patient statements which present the vision of the patients without perceptible distortion. Porter (1987b:34) says of the history of the distrust of what mental patients have to say:

> From the nineteenth century onwards, organic theories permitted a deafness to what the mad said, a deafness ironically akin to that indifference to communication which mad people themselves allegedly betrayed. Therapeutics present similar dilemmas. Thus even the advocates of 'moral therapy' . . . were not interested in listening to what the mad had to say for themselves, or in direct, person-to-person verbal communication. They were preoccupied instead with what might be called 'behaviorist' techniques of rendering their speech proper.

Strauss, et al. (1964:263) indicate that it is necessary to forget that psychiatric patients are psychiatric cases in order to see them as persons who are capable of facing the hospital, their internal life in it, and the facts of their own illnesses: "Patients, like other human beings, are able to participate in any of the social processes which are usually found in hospitals." No less a figure in world psychiatry than William A. White (*in* Grob 1985:92) says that the testimony of psychiatric patients can and should be accepted in courts of law:

> [M]any patients are perfectly well able to give testimony, in fact quite as able to give testimony as persons of sound mind; and I may say that many of them are better able to give testimony than are many people who have not been adjudicated. The idea that because a person's testimony is clear and coherent and to the point that therefore he is not suffering from mental disease . . . is only based upon complete misinformation or rather lack of information regarding the mental state of those who are mentally ill.

We may begin to present the data and test the possibilities of testimony, not legal but social, by the patients. At the same time, in the process of evaluating the statements, it seems to me that it is necessary to realize that in the interviews some patients would surely have been conscious that their responses, possibly, might be passed along to the medical staff; so they may have considered their own presentations of themselves and given them personal directions, as a way of communicating with their doctors. This does not detract but rather adds to their value. Contradictions are also found, not only within single responses but also in the associations brought out by different questions. But, certainly, contradiction, as a frank acknowledgment of ambivalence or as parapraxis, does not distinguish mental patients from the rest of humanity. We will see all of this in the materials to be presented.

As an introduction to the data, in consequence of my interest in patients' opinions of the atmosphere of the pavilion itself and their contentment there, I asked them two successive questions: 42, "How do you like Pavilion 20 in general?," and 43, "Are you satisfied or not? If not, why?" In evaluating their responses it will be well to remember that these are charity patients speaking, poor people in a poor country, many of whom were living in marginal circumstances (inadequate shelter, overcrowding, no toilets, no electicity, no running water, no garbage disposal, and so on), if they were not street people.[2] The patients answered:

> Patient Aguila[3]: 42. I like it because it's large. It's well

ventilated. I like the care by the doctors and the nurses. Also the radio with its loudspeakers, which has made for a pleasant atmosphere. Then, as for the patients, there are a good number of them with whom I rub elbows in a friendly way. Since they have games, chess, checkers, and other parlor games, for those people who are in condition to play them it's something to do. They find comfort and distraction which benefits their spirits a great deal, improving some and making it possible for others to pass their time.

43. I'm satisfied, sure, because of my condition as a convalescent. I'm getting the care that increases that satisfaction, happiness, and contentment. It's possible for me to go home regularly on Saturdays and come back to the pavilion on Tuesday mornings. That's why I'm satisfied.

Patient Borja: 42. It's one of the best here in the Hospital. It's the most modern, the one with the greatest comfort. I mean, from the point of view that it's free.

43. They brought me here against my will. I'm not satisfied. It's not my kind of place.

Patient Cabral: 42. As a new pavilion, there's plenty in it that's new and advanced. Really, there's good care, as much by the doctors as by the nurses.

43. I don't have any complaint about anyone. I don't have any enemies, I think, and I get along well with everybody. That's why I'm satisfied.

Patient Chocano: 42. This pavilion is a modern, comfortable one, well ventilated, with enough light and cleanliness. With enough comfort, it could be said. They even give us the luxury of having vegetable gardens. And it could be said that it looks like a crystal palace, with its modern dining room, even though it doesn't have a good chef. Well, what are we going to do!

43. [This question was not asked.]

Patient Dejo: 42. I like the patio it has, the gardens, the benches for sitting, the nice view.

43. Well, sure.

Patient Estrada: 42. Well, it's good. That's all.

43. Yes.

Patient Flores: 42. I don't like it. Jail is never pleasant.

43. [This question was not asked.]

Patient Gálvez: 42. All the care they take is all right for the most part. I can't say it's good. The pavilion is a bit large. It's big enough to move around in and its bathrooms are nearly clean.
43. Yes, I'm satisfied.

Patient Huerta: 42. It's a modern and comfortable pavilion. But you can see that the way they handle the food is deficient. Also, the attendants are uncultured. They are people who aren't prepared to work in a hospital like this one.
43. As for being content, no. I have to adapt to it and improve till I can leave and go to work for my five children. As for the doctors and nurses, all right. But not the attendants, no, because they sometimes throw out the food they refuse to give a person.

Patient Iglesias: 42. It's very pretty, very pleasant. It offers good health.
43. Yes.

Patient Justo: 42. I like it just the way it is, the way it operates.
43. Yes, I'm satisfied.

Patient Lora: 42. It's the newest pavilion. It has its bathrooms, attendants, radio, music, newspapers.
43. I want to leave. I'm anxious to leave so I can see what I can do outside. I want to forget I've been sick.

Patient Llerena: 42. I don't like it. I'm here temporarily.
43. I'm at peace, and naturally so because my personality is like that.

Patient Márquez: 42. Let there be a lot of harmony here.
43. I'm quite satisfied. I've improved a lot.

Patient Negrín: 42. It seems to me that it's quite large, with a lot of ventilation. There's a big patio where the air circulates. I think that's very good. There's not enough ventilation in the dormitories.
43. I want to leave. I want to go out.

Patient Ñeco: 42. Good. It's very good here.
43. I'm satisfied, happy, content. I haven't left for home, and that's the fault of my brothers. They're careless.

Patient Ortiz: 42. I like it because it's very hygienic and there's a lot of space. It's very clean.

43. Yes, I'm satisfied. I have a better time than anybody.

Patient Peña: 42. It's elegant.

43. I'd like to go out and walk in the street.

Patient Quintana: 42. I like it because it's a modern construction.

43. Yes, but I'm worried about personal things. There's nobody to help me.

Patient Reyes: 42. I like the whole group of fellows.

43. Yes, with reservations about the pills and the inconvenience.

Patient Salas: [The interview had ended prematurely.]

Patient Tapia: 42. I like it that everyone is respectful, friendly, and proper in what they do.

43. For now, well, I'm satisfied.

Patient Ureta: 42. You must see that it's a pavilion that was recently built. It's modern. So I'm not afraid to try it out and find out how well we're getting on.

43. I'm at peace. Yes, I'm satisfied.

Patient Villa: 42. I don't want to be here a long time. I'm ready to leave.

43. I'm all right. They treat me well. I just want to get out.

Patient Yáñez: 42. It's good. It has a good patio for moving around in, for conversing with the other patients.

43. Yes, but now I'm a little bit upset because I'd like to spend a month with my family.

Patient Zevallos: 42. Do you mean the life here or the state of our mind? It's a very large pavilion where you can get better treatment. The other pavilions are closed in. This one has its effects on the patients. The doctors know what kind of treatment a person needs.

43. Why wouldn't I be satisfied?

Patient Armas: 42. I don't like it. It's suitable for people who have money, rich ones. What is suitable for poor people like us is Pavilion 4.

43. [This question was not asked.]

Feeding was one of the most urgent problems for the patients of a charity service. They expressed themselves very well on these matters in their responses to the question, 45. "How do you like the food?":

> Patient Aguila: Well, in that sense, it's a difficult thing. At home-- Here we have a menu that is healthy and pleasant. [He laughs and straightens his body on the seat.] There are always foods I don't like, but I have to eat them. What I miss is the fruit because that was my habit. I'm a fruit eater.
>
> Patient Borja: I don't like the food. It's very bad.
>
> Patient Cabral: It's often good, it's often bad. It depends on a person's taste.
>
> Patient Chocano: I've always liked food. I've liked it good, as a good son of X_____ [he names a European country from which his father moved to Peru]. But what they give us is quite nutritious and healthy. It might be that in time it will be better.
>
> Patient Dejo: I don't like it. Every day there are beans, and beans.
>
> Patient Estrada: It's good, pleasant, and nutritious.
>
> Patient Flores: It's bad. We never eat meat. It's insipid.
>
> Patient Gálvez: As for the food, well, it ought to be a little bit more flavored. The meat and the noodles don't have any flavoring. I like salad, eggs, milk, but there's none of that.
>
> Patient Huerta: Sometimes it's good and sometimes it's bad. It depends.
>
> Patient Iglesias: It's very tasty.
>
> Patient Justo: For me, from the point of view that I'm not sick, it seems to me that it ought to be a little better, the kind I can't get because I'm here in the Hospital. But it's healthy. Beginning with breakfast, this is what we get: they give us a breakfast that seems to me far from being better, because when we have milk it's very strange, very much watered down. They give us black coffee with

two pieces of bread all week. Then, at lunch, we have what's called the second. You have to swallow it as well as you can. They don't give us meat. When they give us meat they serve it in very small portions, so that it seems to me that we're always hungry. Once in a while we get good lunches in which there's plenty of meat.

Patient Lora: It's not the kind of food I get at home. They keep giving the same foods. That's annoying. Family cooking doesn't exist here. But my appetite's good.

Patient Llerena: You have to tolerate the food, because if you don't take advantage of it, it works against your health.

Patient Márquez: Good. It's better food.

Patient Negrín: I don't eat here. My mother brings lunch for me.

Patient Ñeco: It's good, all right, enough to fill the stomach.

Patient Ortiz: I like it. For me, everything's good. There's no bad food. The garbanzos are very tasty. Chocano fixes onions and *ají* [hot pepper which chopped with the onions, both from the garden, makes a garnish (*salsa*) to liven the bland Hospital food]. Very tasty.

Patient Peña: It's the same that they bring every day.

Patient Quintana: It's not good. I don't like it. It's not prepared well. They give us tea or coffee in the morning without milk.

Patient Reyes: How could I tell you? The food's all right.

Patient Tapia: I like clean food with pleasant seasoning.

Patient Ureta: Let it be well cooked and palatable.

Patient Villa: Good.

Patient Yáñez: For example, there should be good milk and hot bread at breakfast. Sometimes the milk is bad and the bread is stale.

Patient Zevallos: It's something we don't pay for. That's the way it should be. The food is enough for getting better.

> Patient Armas: I'd like it better if it were well prepared. I like everything. The cooks are all right. Some days it's good and other days it's bad.

Another problem for patients was how to fill time during the long, days, weeks, months, and years of patienthood. Although game equipment existed, it was possible to organize sports, and there were reading materials in the pavilion, I observed that many patients spent their time walking in their personal territories next to the walls or, simply, sitting down doing nothing. One of the most impressive characteristics of Pavilion 20 was the sparse social interaction to be found there. Indeed, one of my greatest difficulties in getting used to research tasks was the relative silence and social coldness of the place.[4] An extract from my observational notes of September 14, at 11 in the morning in the commons room, reveals this low level of group activity:

> It seems to me that this unit is constructed so that people who don't want to have contacts don't have to have them. Interaction is at a minimum. Right now there are only two patients dancing to radio music in here. They try to get a third to join them and he breaks away abruptly. Then they break up themselves. Also, T_____ and V_____, across the way, are talking. This is all the visible interaction I can see. It is clear that others notice what is going on, so we might conceive of an inner interaction here. F_____ comes over to sit down next to me and ask for another cigarette. He says to me: "Who would God be?" I answer: "It's not known." He nods, sits for a while, and then gets up to leave. I wonder whether a unit like this is built to cut down on interaction? And, likewise, if a different arrangement--say, smaller with benches placed so that people could interact more easily, and even engage in group activities--would have any negative function, considering what they are trying to accomplish here?
>
> I realized the other day that patients don't know each other's names, or at least many names. I asked V_____ what was D_____'s name and he couldn't answer. However, R_____ knows it and possibly has a wider acquaintance. Last week, V_____ excused his poor knowledge of doctors' and nurses' names by saying he'd only been here a few weeks.

The answer to my puzzlement over the discrepancy between physical arrangements and psychiatric goals turned out to be that when Pavilion 20 was built the psychiatric staff, having had no input to the architects, had to accept the physical plant the way it was and adapt to it as best they could. Of course, people who want to be together can overcome physical obstacles. But these patients did not. Bockoven (1972:31) points out that the "very essence of mental illness . . . is an incapacity to get along with other people." Since the character of the pavilion was a schizophrenic one, Falloon's (1988:129) comment on schizophrenia and the breakdown of social skills is most relevant:

> Schizophrenia, in both the acute and subacute phases, is associated with a wide range of impairments in perception and information-processing. In the acute phase of schizophrenia the patients' ability to interpret social cues may be severely distorted by delusional perception. Behavior that would commonly engender a positive connotation of friendship or acceptance, such as a smile, a head nod, a pat on the back, or a handshake, may be interpreted quite differently by floridly deluded persons. Such gestures may be considered to have a sinister, threatening, or special meaning that is idiosyncratic to the persons suffering from the delusion. The patients' subsequent social response to such cues is, therefore, likely to be considered inappropriate--at times bizarre--and lead to rejection and the breakdown of social relationships.

Social withdrawal[5] can be seen in the interview materials from Pavilion 20. In response to the question, 32, "How are the patients, how do they treat you?," the patients said:

> Patient Aguila: There's a good number of them plainly getting better, which makes them sociable and friendly. I haven't had any kind of trouble here.
>
> Patient Borja: I never have anything to do with them.
>
> Patient Cabral: The patients, generally, I think that I don't have any enemy among the patients according to the way they treat me. You notice when a patient doesn't care for you, and this hasn't happened since I've been in this pavilion.
>
> Patient Chocano: There's a majority who are readapting and improving notably, things which they seem to achieve from the example of other patients who lead a moderate and peaceful life. Still, there are some who persist in their abnormalities and acquired vices. And that's due largely to their own state of ignorance the the

quality of the life they've led. They seem to be improving because many of them are getting used to the atmosphere here.

Patient Dejo: They are calm. They treat me well in every way.

Patient Estrada: Good. There are some who are disturbed because they're a bit sensitive, but most of them are having a great improvement in the illness that they're suffering.

Patient Flores: Well, we know what a patient is. I have very little to do with them, almost nothing.

Patient Gálvez: Some are a little annoying. With others you have to keep away from them for a while. They all have their bad times. They behave themselves.

Patient Huerta: They're all my friends. I haven't had any trouble here.

Patient Iglesias: They're very sick. Yes, they're very sick and so they don't have anything to do with me.

Patient Justo: The patients are situated on patients' terrain. They don't depart from the limits which enclose them or mark them. In any case they behave themselves like patients asking for a cure, and staying well like that.

Patient Lora: I'd like to be able--- I can't always get to know them. There are some who are very well known, like C_____ who always escapes naked. There are some, two or three--- I haven't made many friends. I know T_____ who is a great conversationalist. I don't go up to him to talk but to find out what's going on in his newspapers. There's another boy, too. I haven't made friends.

Patient Llerena: I have to be understanding and tolerant with them often, because with so many companions or friends you just have to get along.

Patient Márquez: Good. They don't have respect. They have more respect for the person of the one who offers them the most gratification.

Patient Negrín: The patients seem calm, just so. A few of them behave extravagantly. They don't behave themselves as a person should behave. A few of them are like that.

Patient Ñeco: In the best way. I don't deal with any of them. I treat them with respect so that they can respect me.

Patient Ortiz: Good. There aren't any abusive people here. Everybody's good.

Patient Peña: Just good.

Patient Quintana: They are all sick patients.

Patient Reyes: They're all right.

Patient Tapia: They're--- They are respectful to you, and some of them are friendly.

Patient Ureta: As for the patients, there are some whom one can trust, but they all treat me well.

Patient Villa: There are some who are good, friendly, sincere.

Patient Yáñez: There are some who are very good friends because they like to converse or play games. Some are angry and can harm you. Some don't want to have much to do with the others.

Patient Zevallos: Everybody behaves well. They like me. There are always some who don't.

Patient Armas: They're good. We talk. Sometimes they ask me to join them. I'd be delegate for physical culture if they'd ask me. But I'm tired of organizations. Now there's one forming, a sporting organization. Last night they invited me to join them.

I asked this group of patients a series of sociometric questions about their friendships (33 and 34), dormitory companions (35), dining companions (36), companions in games and sports (37), and with whom they would choose to go out on a day's leave (38). In response to the last item, of the 26 interviews, 10 named different invididuals in the pavilion (although one of them said, "With what's his name, [and after a pause] with P_____."), while 10 named members of their families, and 6 said that they would prefer to go on leave alone. To the question on companions in games and sports, of 24 subjects questioned, 10 named different persons in the pavilion, 7 said "nobody" or "I don't play," and 7 responses were evasive. Their responses to the question which dealt with table companions indicated that they knew best other patients they shared food with: of the 24 subjects asked the question, 18 named individuals, 1 (Patient Llerena) said, "There aren't any, because I sit where there's an unoccupied bench," and 5 gave evasive replies like "I work, I take care of them, I'm the first one in the pantry to serve them," "I don't have a permanent table," "We're-- I don't remember who they are became we're not friends," "There are four of us but I've forgotten their names," or simply "I don't remember."

A series of questions forming a bridge between feelings about being patients and conceptions of the patient role were: 63, "What happened to you when you came to the Hospital, to Pavilion 20?"; 64, "What things do you consider most important for getting used to it?"; 65, "What were your greatest difficulties in getting used to it?"; and 66, "Supposing I were a new patient who had just come, what advice would you give me to get used to it more quickly?"

> Patient Aguila: 63. I remember that it was possible for me to ask the doctors if my treatment could be as an outpatient. I could do that because it cost me a lot of work to get used to being hospitalized. I was very lonely for my family and because I never had been hospitalized--- I was used to engaging in sports, going to the libraries. I have many relatives in Lima whom I'm used to visiting, and even my friends. Later, when my electroshock treatment was over, the simple fact of walking around the same place for 24 hours was intolerable. Then, from the doctors' orders I knew that in my case I needed lots of rest, completely to stop worrying about all the unpleasant things. They gave me confidence by making me see that my improvement depended, above all, on me, on my exercising control over my attitudes and showing sincerely the symptoms I experienced during the treatment. What I remember most was that restlessness at the end of the electroshock treatment. Yes, earlier I felt strong grief. And then a great relief grew. It had been a generalized grief that came over me. As a consequence my bad humor was a kind of contamination of everything. One is bitter and it gets generalized to everything. It was like I was heavily loaded, and then I was surprised by the immense tranquility that came to me. I was so surprised that I told the doctors. I went to the window to

look out, and I liked it. They let me walk in the patio. . . . I hope I can get out soon. The social worker is helping me look for work.

64. Making friends. Then--- I think that's the only factor. Otherwise, you feel lonely. Friends are necessary to have conversations, play chess, talk about the movie they show on Thursdays. They ought to have movies more than once a week. Patients who have improved enough, and who don't have relatives, ought to be able to go outside with the attendants. Maybe in a bus to see the sights. They ought to have magazines in the office, maybe a library. There should be someone to instruct patients in games or group discussions. Cleaning duties are manual, but there should be mental exercises as well.

65. and 66. [These questions were not asked.]

Patient Borja: 63. I was a little uncomfortable. I felt bad. When they gave me an injection for coming here I was at home. A nurse came in and brought me to the Hospital. I remember everything.

64. If they would give me better food.

65. Yes, I had a difficulty. I'm not becoming happy.

66. That this is the best pavilion. It has a very good administrative system. Just that.

Patient Cabral: 63. When I was talking with a patient who was not at all mentally ill, I was afraid, wondering if I were sick or not. Rather, I had doubts, I was shocked, I didn't know. That was my first impression in my first conversation, and I didn't feel equal to that patient. And I asked myself why I had come, what I had. Then the doctor made me understand that it was from an alcoholic infection and that I had to get cured.

64. I noticed that things were not like I thought. The fear from before went away and I realized that it wasn't like a jail but like a clinic, a hospital, which is the general word for a place where there's medical care.

65. [This question was not asked.]

66. The advice I'd give you is, first, to take you around the hospital, introduce you to some of the other patients, and teach you about the life that goes on in the hospital. And also to make you understand that it's not what a person imagines.

Patient Chocano: 63. I almost don't remember about the first time. It's like vaguely remembering a nightmare, something that isn't worth the trouble, because now I'm feeling completely well and normal. And I can claim that and show it everywhere. The doctor who has observed me and followed closely the process of my reestablishment will testify to it. It seems to me that I felt sicker than I was. That's very natural when you find yourself in the midst of really sick people, as I believed and soon found out. It's like that with many of them, in spite of the doctors' efforts. That must be because the disease is deeply rooted or the lesion is very serious. Although they have improved a lot by now, they aren't cured. . . .

64. It seems that now that I'm feeling better I don't want to continue staying here any more. If I go back to the society in which I've lived, to the world of work in which I've always participated, I may be useful to my family. I'd like to work in commercial activity, which I've done since I was small. I'm still thinking of making a home and living a new life.

65. The change of atmosphere even affects plants, as is quite natural. I've slipped and at the beginning it was hard for me to adapt to conditions, since here everything is different. However, because I believe that man is a creature of habits, readaptation to the world of the living will be easy.

66. This isn't a pessimistic resignation but quite to the contrary a healthy optimism, a solid faith in the complete cure from my disturbance, my mental disequilibrium, or my sickness, however you want to call it, and having the most complete conficence that I will come out well and completely cured. Many of those who come here are overwhelmed by thinking at first that there are so many who've been here for so many years. And there's a reason. It's quite right that it makes them think that way. But you have to throw out those ideas, because out on the streets there are possibly more sick people, if it may be said like that. Nevertheless, inside this hospital, its means of living allow them not to have to deal in such a glaring way with their character as really sick people.

Patient Dejo: 63. I was vexed. I didn't sleep. That's why I came.

64. Nothing. Now I'm getting used to it. Well, I've been here for a year and a half.

65. None.

66. So that they would get along with you? You should have patience. When your treatment is over, they'll give you leave to go outside. That's all.

Patient Estrada: 63. I felt sick and my mother brought me. . . .

64. Just resigning yourself.

65. It wasn't hard to get used to it because I'd been a patient here

before. The first time it seemed a bit strange, weird, but later I got used to it.

66. You should obey the the rules and the discipline of the Hospital.

Patient Flores: 63. There was pressure, torture. How terrible a person feels when he finds he is a prisoner! It's something that can't be told.

64. This is not ever going to happen. It's just freedom. With freedom you can get everything. Dr. Fernández told me, "You don't have any clothing and there's no place for you outside."

65. [This question was not asked.]

66. You should resign yourself and conform. You can't give advice because everybody feels the same.

Patient Gálvez: 63. I felt a little weak. It was my mind. My temples hurt and I was a little tired.

64. You have to have a little patience.

65. The only thing was being face to face.

66. You should have a little patience, peacefulness, and good manners. And also to get together with the good ones. They're not all the same, and some of them are aggressive, half crazy. They have their degree of culture. You can't be friends with everybody.

Patient Huerta: 63. Sincerely, I was quite shocked to find myself in a hospital like this one, where I never expected to be in my life. . . .

64. Being in harmony with the doctors, my wife, the children, my mother.

65. At the beginning you aren't used to it. Some of them are here eight years and then they don't ever want to leave.

66. That your treatment's going to be short, that you won't be here a long time. That's what I'd do, because although it seems like a lie, it's easier to get better for somebody without a family.

Patient Iglesias: 63. I felt physically exhausted.

64. I was in good health.

65. Finding myself with sick people.

66. You should look for friends.

Patient Justo: 63. When they brought me I felt quite well. I could have been a little sick, but when they brought me I was better. That's the way it happened. I woke up from sleeping and when they told me

I didn't move. They told me that they'd brought me in an ambulance. Later they gave me an insulin treatment.

64. With regard to psychological functions-- In the case of being in the Hospital, I'd like to be married because it's no exaggeration, but not being like that I go along with what's called onanism, because I'm not sick. I'd like to marry a woman nurse and work as a male nurse. That's why I'm trying to see, in case I remain in the Hospital. I'd like to marry a girl who's an assistant here.

65. The idea that I wasn't mentally ill. I was horribly depressed when I faced being in the Hospital. That was the greatest difficulty.

66. Avoid looking a lot at the patients, because you discover many things in them which amount to the greatest horrors which, when they appear, aren't even seen in any war. I say this not because I was thinking of being an army officer in 1945, but I couldn't get into the Chorrillos school [the Peruvian military academy]. Later I worked in two social causes, and I was dismissed from both unjustly, liquidated in a bad manner. Since I didn't find work, then, I understood that both employees and laborers--because I worked in the first one as a laborer--suffered a lot. So I wanted to be a professional, but since I didn't have the resources to get a higher education, I wanted to be a public accountant. I began to read for it in the library in S_____, and I finished in Lima. I wanted to be an army officer, but I couldn't because they brought me here. Even a patient doesn't get used to the horrors of the patients here, especially a professional who doesn't have a profession and who stays in relation to the mental illnesses of the Hospital. That's why for a patient's getting used to it in Pavilion 20, I'd advise you not to look at the horrors there are in the patients. Not too long ago they told me that a patient had died, and I was afraid that I'd die. Then I thought it would be better not to think about such horrors.

Patient Lora: 63. [This question was not asked.]

64. I'm afraid of getting used to it. I don't want to. The Hospital Larco Herrera has its paying patients, but we're not that and I reject it. To get used to it would be dangerous.

65. Psychiatry ought to be a copy of life outside, so that the patient wouldn't lose responsibility.

66. All kinds of patients come here, some who need special treatment and some whose families take care of them better. I'd ask you what things bother you the most. There are some who rebel against the idea of being mental patients. Some have prejudices and others accept their state. The doctor observes and reveals. To be cured, a patient has to recognize his faults, his illness. It's necessary

to listen to the doctors.

Patient Llerena: 63. Here, a while ago, I had a dose of serpasol and it changed my nature automatically, in my movements and in the loss of my memory.

64. Inside the Hospital I don't think that there are private resources like being free. There are things, according to the food, the clothing. As for the rest, the purpose, for example, is recreation.

65. On occasion, the food. Then the personal confinement and the unpaid cooperation.

66. I'd advise you to keep your wits about you, to get along better. Then good will while you're here, according to medical orders, in order to recover your condition like the rest.

Patient Márquez: 63. I felt quite dizzy.

64. Just the work.

65. When I couldn't find union with another person.

66. I'd put you in touch with everything, and if you were without some things I'd show them to you. I'd tell you to be more peaceful, to get along better, not to be too friendly, and to respect the nurses.

Patient Negrín: 63. I was sick with something going on in my shoulder. I got better here. . . .

64. Here life is peaceful. It's easy to be here, away from the noise of the city, the responsibilities.

65. The only shock I had was insulin. It's hard to be in bed so much, because it makes a person weak. They take your clothes away from you. That makes you ashamed.

66. Just that you should be at peace, have patience, and try to observe the rest of the patients. That would be good advice.

Patient Ñeco: 63. I felt bad, sick, a very offensive man. You wouldn't have spoken to me.

64. I don't want to stay here. I don't ask anybody for anything, not even a match.

65. There wasn't any problem. Nothing happens to a man who's a good worker. I don't have anything to do with anybody.

66. That you be patient, that you'd get your freedom soon. It's necessary to submit to treatment.

Patient Ortiz: 63. I felt bad. I was disturbed. They called me "Superman." I was fighting a lot and I lost my teeth from being hit. I suffered a lot. I could write a history of my life here and they could make a movie there in the United States.

What I needed was to have patience, to help the attendants clean the pavilion, to cooperate, to keep on the alert and tell when they want to escape.

65. I got used to it when I came. What are you going to do? The Hospital was like a paradise. I got used to it, like at home.

66. Have patience, wait because you're going to get well soon, make friends, and have a good character.

Patient Peña: 63. I felt somewhat sick in my head. Before that I was working where I was living and my head was all right.

64. I don't know.

65. I don't know.

66. You have to have patience and then it will be all right.

Patient Quintana: 63. I was completely sad, very sad, because I'd left home.

64. Having a good life, good health, the work life. I was working as en employee. I'd like to be an employee here.

65. I was like the rest in the beginning. It was the lack of habit because I'd been admitted recently.

66. Behave yourself with all of them, don't fight, be good with the nurses and the patients, just that.

Patient Reyes: 63. I felt well.

64. [This question was not asked.]

65. The treatments, the pills and injections.

66. Just that you get used to insulin treatments.

Patient Tapia: 63. I was feeling something in understanding.

64. That what you're doing is in good order.

65. The study of professional categories.

66. I'd let you know what you don't know, for example, how much time you'll be here, and that you be friendly and moderate, just that.

Patient Ureta: 63. When my family brought me, I don't remember well, but little by little my memory cleared up. They put me on insulin.

64. The food and the rest for the body that they give you.

65. When I came to and looked around, what I saw was that the doctor was curing the other patients. That gave me a little scare. When I saw them giving electroshock to P_____, when I was the first

one in the room, it shook me quite a lot.

66. I'd tell you to have a peaceful life this way, that you keep in mind all the doctor's orders, the same with the nurses. That's the way to have a peaceful life.

Patient Villa: 63. I don't remember.

64. I want to get out of here. How am I going to get used to it?

65. It was the time for going to bed. You have to do it. It's the same when you get up, when the attendant says so.

66. It's just according to a person's character, and just looking at his behavior. I don't remember anything more.

Patient Yáñez: 63. I felt strange. I didn't know anybody.

64. You get used to what there is here, but it's not like at home. It ought to be more like it is at home so a person would get used to it.

65. Well, for example, at home I had friends. I could have a conversation or go to the movies. Here I didn't have friends. There wasn't anybody to talk to or play games with.

66. You should try to make friends among the patients in good condition here, and play games to pass the time here, just that.

Patient Zevallos: 63. They brought me--I didn't come!--because I was in a clinic, disturbed, without any peace. Here, little by little, I got rid of the bad thoughts I had, and now the doors of my life are open. It's something very serious for patients who are suffering from nerves. The noise of downtown isn't for the best rest of patients who suffer in their minds.

64. Having strength, and good will, and enduring everything we see here. As long as I have my five senses, there isn't anything that's hard.

65. When I was sick, maybe I had problems, but now my situation is all right and I can bear anything. It can be complicated when you think about problems.

66. Give good food to a patient, advice directed at the person, for example, to behave yourself with everybody, to get along, and to tell the doctor everything you feel, everything that happens to you, like irritation. That is, I'd be your friend right away, and do anything I could for you, so that you'd have the confidence to tell the true way you feel. I'd help you with treatments, too. There are many times when a patient is afraid to tell the truth to the doctor, or he believes that the doctor can do something to him.

Patient Armas: 63. My mind was broken. That should be explained. It was my fault. I had a lot of women, many sexual relations.

64. That they don't throw us out but, rather, treat us well. I'd have gone home, but they treat me well and I've stayed.

65. [This question was not asked.]

66. The only thing is that you should behave himself so they can treat you the best way.

A response which is very revealing of the definition of the patient's role is answer to the question, 41, "What is the patient's duty?" Unfortunately, it was not included in the schedule given to the first twelve patients; here is what the others said:

Patient Llerena: The patient is the sick person whose health requires attention in order to recover normal stability. It's a matter of his being inside the society. That jurisdiction should be respected.

Patient Márquez: They have to have a lot of common sense to take care of the patient. They have to have a lot of responsibility, give help, and have something of affection and patience for what a patient can do.

Patient Negrín: He should keep observing what effect the medicine has on him, and he should try to talk with the doctor about his case.

Patient Ñeco: Respect. He ought to be respectful to the nurse, to the doctor. He should do his work: sweeping, bringing water. Naturally, respect and work. It's nothing big, being respectful and a worker.

Patient Ortiz: Patients don't do anything. They should help. They should take care of the plants. Most of them are very ungrateful. They eat, sleep, and they don't do anything to help. T_____ is a good person. He works.

Patient Peña: He should mind the nurses.

Patient Quintana: He should behave himself with the male nurses, and with the women nurses, too. He should be friendly to everybody, agreeable, and do no harm. That's all.

Patient Reyes: He should ask about the treatment.

Patient Tapia: He should behave with respect, be friendly, and accept their professional activities.

Patient Ureta: He should be frank with his doctor and keep him up to date about all the diseases he has, so that the doctor can cure them.

Patient Yáñez: He should behave himself with the attendants, and not be impulsive with the nurses, and also with the doctor.

Patient Zevallos: What a person should do is act to help in the doctor's treatment, so that the doctor can come to find out how he is suffering.

Patient Armas: He should behave himself as best he can in everything connected with our stay here.

The questions, 61, "What is a hospital like Víctor Larco Herrera?" and 62, "Have your ideas changed after coming here?, how?, what expectation did you have?", were designed to get at the concepts the patients had about mental hospitals (what I now refer to as "hospital image"). The patients' responses add much to the picture we are developing:

Patient Aguila: 61. I never had occasion to think about something like that. I knew that medical specialists in these diseases existed, and that it was possible that patients might get well. That was all I thought. I was afraid. This fear diminished little by little.
62. [This question was not asked.]

Patient Borja: 61. It's a place where they cure patients.
62. No.

Patient Cabral: 61. It's a hospital for all kinds of mental illnesses, curable and incurable. It depends on the case.
62. [This question was not asked.]

Patient Chocano: 61. This is thought of the best hospital for mental patients exclusively in the whole country. For its location, its excellent climate, the good distribution of its pavilions, its competent administration, its good plan of specialized measures, and the good auxilliary personnel of nurses.
62. Of course. They have indeed changed. Now I'm convinced that it's no longer merely a matter of an insane asylum or a place for

seclusion, but it's a modern hospital, a well managed one. Lack of trust, quite rightly so of course, comes from what one doesn't understand.

Patient Dejo: 61. It's a hospital for mental patients, ones who can't sleep. It's for idiots, too. That's all.

62. I felt strange here looking at patients who were out of their minds. I think the same as before, When I came here, I came the way I am now. I couldn't sleep at night. I had nervous attacks. I was vexed.

Patient Estrada: 61. It's a hospital for mental patients.

62. I don't think so.

Patient Flores: 61. There isn't another one here. There are others, but they are private.

62. I don't understand you.

Patient Gálvez: 61. It's a hospital which has enough conveniences for the patient's rest, the mental patient. It's for rest and cure.

62. Not at all. I've been completely well.

Patient Huerta: 61. It's a hospital for the treatment and cure of mental illnesses.

62. I was already here and I didn't believe my illness was---that the treatment might not be very long. Now I guess it's going to be three or four months. So how long will it be?

Patient Iglesias: 61. Where they take care of nervous patients.

62. I never had ideas about the Hospital.

Patient Justo: 61. It's a place where patients with mental illnesses are brought for their recovery or cure.

62. No.

Patient Lora: 61. It's an establishment whose purpose is to be a guide for the development of the human mind. This is an ideal. But there are people who have internal conflicts which require professional advice to clear up these things that lead to disturbances. The individual becomes normal. He acquires everything. It's for throwing light on the shadows. It's what ought to be. There are people who aren't sick but who could get sick and need help in order to keep their clarity.

62. The fear is because what the person is called outside is "crazy." He's afraid and he calls himself "crazy." And this gives us our idea of what a hospital is like. Now I have a bigger idea of what it is. Some are incurable, or the treatment is very difficult. Maybe they're curable. I understand the reality better.

Patient Llerena: 61. Here in Peru there are societies like what I've known since I was very small.

62. I'm like what *La Crónica* [a Lima newspaper] published last Sunday about rehabilitated people. So maybe I think of myself as rehabilitated, but I wouldn't be inside a hospital.

Patient Márquez: 61. There are more authorities in this Hospital.

62. Well, sure. I'm thinking about what I used to be, before.

Patient Negrín: 61. They try to cure mental illness with insulin treatments, and electroshock.

62. I never worried about it. Frankly, I was afraid of going in. It seemed to me that I was going to be isolated. I thought of a mentally ill person as one who didn't understand anything.

Patient Ñeco: 61. It's a sanatorium, where they cure patients.

62. I forgot all kinds of things. When I came, I didn't know anything. Now I'm healthy.

Patient Ortiz: 61. It's a teaching hospital where they prepare doctors and nurses. It's a school.

62. No.

Patient Peña: 61. I don't know.

62. I don't know.

Patient Quintana: 61. It's shelter for all the patients. It's like a hospice where patients are cured and go out in good health.

62. No, nothing.

Patient Reyes: 61. It's a hospital for taking care of the crazy people, isn't it?

62. [This question was not asked.]

Patient Tapia: 61. It's a degree of profession which gives people's voluntary good will.

62. So, now my fundamental principles are established.

Patient Ureta: 61. It's a hospital where all the mental patients are.
62. No, because I've also seen it.

Patient Villa: 61. I don't know much about that.
62. I don't remember.

Patient Yáñez: 61. It's a place where they take care of patients who are suffering some kind of mental or cerebral alteration.
62. No, they're the same as what I thought before.

Patient Zevallos: 61. It's made for the purpose of treating mental illnesses, especially, and giving the patient the best treatment that can be given. That's the reason why the doctors specialize in this Hospital.
62. I don't know completely.

Patient Armas: 61. It's a place where poor people gather to have themselves cured for charity, without charge. There's board for those with money. It belongs to the Lima Public Charity Society.
62. [This question was not asked.]

However, it turned out that much more revealing patient responses were those that dealt with their role expectations of Hospital personnel. These were of value not only in the sense of providing a more extense and complete picture of their hospital images, but also in the sense of uncovering something more of their feelings and conceptions. I asked them several questions about the doctors, of which the most useful were: 13, "What would you like to receive from the doctors?", 14, "How would you like them to treat you?", 15, "What is good in the doctors and what is bad?", and 16, "What would be ideal?". I present here only a selection of the responses that I believe are pertinent to the goals I have outlined:

Patient Cabral: 13. Often, I believe, the doctor would have to tell the patient about his case, that he has found out the illness he has, and more or less the time he has to stay in the hospital. This would be to pacify the patient's morale. . . . In all of that, often, there turns out to be a kind of disaccord betwen the patient and the doctor, when the patient doesn't know the reality, and he begins to think about things that, frankly, are unreal. That's not good for the patient. So, often, escape takes place because they don't know what they have and they are afraid they're going to be in the Hospital all their lives. That's why most of them are thinking about escape.

14. It's according to the illness they have. It depends on them. Often the patient doesn't have to say much and he's at his doctor's orders. The doctors don't even know what a person has. They don't say. You have to depend on the doctor, who decides about the illness that he thinks you have. Doctors can't handle the quantity of patients that there are in the pavilion. So they talk with their patients once or twice a week. A doctor gives enough time when he comes, but maybe he comes once a week or once every two weeks. The attention relieves patients a lot, because they know that the more attention is given them the sooner discharge is going to happen, and the patients will get out. One thing I don't understand is that there are so many patients who are interned in this hospital because they're alcoholics or mental patients, and they give them daily injections. I think that the hospital could do that with outpatients, instead of internal ones, because, according to the case, you're unhappy being in the hospital away from your family, and often they don't understand you. With mental patients, they feel isolated, and so it can harm them instead of doing them good. . . . Sometimes the doctors don't understand why a person is outside all afternoon. Sometimes it's hard to find companions inside, people to talk to, because a person can't read all the time. They call a person in the morning and they introduce him to someone, and they tell them to be friends. You do that to please the doctor, but you get tired because you can't get along with the illness. The ones who can talk find that it is hard to communicate with those who can't, or those who talk and what they say makes no sense. You put some effort into finding somebody who can talk and understand.

15. What is good is that up to now the doctors who have treated me have tried to make a person out of me. They're tried to advise me and give me good treatment so I'd get well, always giving me a lot of hope that once I left here I wouldn't return. I don't see anything bad in them.

16. It would be to study the foundations, with thorough psychological analyses of the patient.

Patient Chocano: 13. Nothing but the culmination in cure. Of course, it should be beneficial and, if possible, definitive. In a word, to get out completely cured. I think that's desired by all patients.

14. I think it couldn't be done any better.

15. I couldn't say what he might think would be convenient, and, much less, I couldn't suggest to him a method of cure that I don't know about. They almost don't have to do any more than what has

to do with curing, because the matters of cleaning, food, and shelter are already taken care of. They can't change the food that's already ordered by the dietician. The food can't be called either good or bad.

16. That they would try to make life as tolerable as possible, happier, and let us feel the sensation of not being in the condition of people subject to barracks discipline, but, rather, merely at the orders of what ought to exist in a hospital. That's it. There isn't anything else.

Patient Flores: 13. What they could do for me is what they haven't been able to do for 26 years. The doctor told me he was going to look after my case. A year has passed. I went to Dr. Fernández and told him, "Well, a year ago you were going to look after my case." He told me, "Yes, but you have no place to go. There's nothing that can be done." What can you do when they answer you like that? They can't do anything for me. My family brought me here. I asked Dr. Salazar why I was here and how I could get out. He told me, "Behave yourself and then we can visit." I think I'm going to get out when I die. It would be better to die.

14. They can't do anything. Dr. Salazar said it was a matter of authority.

15. All right, they're jailers. Some of them are good but they have you here like a prisoner. It's more worthwhile not to talk to them. It's a matter of opinion. Some are good and others are bad. They can't cure some people. A doctor died one night during an interview.

16. Like I've said to you, if a person can't be cured, how is he going to get well? If one of them died during an interview, how could he cure?

Patient Huerta: That they cure me. What makes me most anxious is to have them cure me, because I have five children, all minors, and there's no one to care for them.

14. Dr. Alba treats me well, as you've just seen. [Dr. Alba has just left us.] I'd like him to treat me in a friendly way, listen to me, solve my case. All married couples fight. My wife hasn't come to see me for ten days. I got married about fifteen years ago. A child was born when she was 14 years old. She had a very sad childhood. I raised the boy and I gave him a good education. The doctor should help me solve these family problems.

15. Logically, the doctors as professionals have to be good. They are specialists in psychiatry. They have to feel for a patient and treat him well.

16. That the patient is cured as rapidly as possible. That would be ideal, that he gets out completely healthy.

Patient Lora: 13. I, for example, my memory is leaving me. It's failing. I don't know, but it would be good if my mind cleared up and they let me out. I'd like to leave for three months but my family is not here. They've come every month, sometimes every two weeks. I've left my studies and the activities I have left are very few. I've never found a job. Now is a good time. But there are prejudices. I'm always going to be afraid of coming back here. The pressures of the university can bring me back again. The doctors tell me that I could go back there, but I don't feel confident of how I would react to the university. I don't want to be a load for my family.

14. They treat me well. Now I'd like to stop talking about illnesses, get out of the hospital, and resume my activities. They always look at you as a patient, or an ex-patient. They're still boys of the same age. That's the part I don't like.

15. If it's so that I would be considered to be sick, let it be a doctor who has treated me often. I'd like the experience. I didn't like electroshock and insulin. I can't talk in public. I lose my ideas. That happened to me once. The doctor treated me for that. The electroshock hurt my back. I've read practical psychology and I've made some suggestions for practice. I had a guilt complex and I began to hurt myself, to burn myself, because I was angry at myself. I let a heavy stone fall on my hand. They can't get those ideas out of me. I'd say that the doctors would be able to do good according to their education and opportunities for study. They have understanding with their education, morale. The bad part would be this: I'm not happy. The doctor does what he wants and the family can't say anything. He can hurt the patient. He doesn't always have patience. That's a matter of personality and character. Sometimes they want to study and they can't cure. The young ones have greater interest and enthusiasm. But that doctor has helped to rid me of a little depression. Doctors have to be special persons with a special character. I can't tell you exactly what they have to be to be good. When they're successful in their specialty they're good. I can't tell you about a bad doctor, except in the case of my tonsil operation. But I don't have documentation, only doubts. I can't spend time here in Larco Herrera easily. They're solicitous here. My relatives come continually to visit and they keep on watching the doctors.

Patient Negrín: 13. I want an explanation of what insulin is in the organism, and the medications they give me so as not to be so blind.

14. Let us have more relations, more visits. Set a time for looking for improvement, and a time to look at the patient and how he's feeling.

15. A real doctor is always with patients, talking with them. I think that this is not true here. A doctor ought to have a deeper understanding.

16. He ought always to be with his patients and try to see how they are getting along, and he should be in touch with the latest advances of science.

Patient Ortiz: 13. That their attention, their way of giving care are good, human. I've received almost all the treatments, sixty-one electroshocks in eleven years and five lumbral punctures. I was in the Hospital Obrero two times and three times here.

14. Affectionately, like the way they're treating me. That's the way they treat mental patients. Otherwise, they wouldn't do them any good.

15. They're all the same. Some are good and some have a violent character. Dr. Gómez is a little violent. Dr. Toro is passive, also Dr. Alba. It's a matter of nature, from too much blood that some of them have.

16. That they are pleasant, passive. That they show the patient joy, friendship, and be pleasant like a father to a son.

Patient Quintana: 13. I'd like to know what the inheritance is that my papa left me. He died in July.

14. To cure my finger, all my external diseases.

15. They right questions they ask you are good. You have to answer as healthily as possible. I can't say what is bad.

16. That all of them always be good, that they help the patient in every way.

Patient Zevallos: 13. The help they are giving me by having me here. They have me here, talking care of me. Blood and bones are worth more than gold.

14. The way they behave, according to the person I am.

15. There are all kinds, good ones and bad ones. It's not good to talk about that if you don't know about it.

16. A doctor ought to be a good person, to know how to deal with all kinds of people, and to know his work.

Patient Armas: 13. That they give us poor people a few more conveniences.

14. I'm not a complainer. I'm happy. I have a great deal of respect and esteem for my bosses because they treat me well.

15. They're good when they have the patience to take care of any request we make. The bad thing is that they don't have enough time to take care of each one of us.

16. It seems to me that it's necessary for them to have a little more interest in the patients, that this would help us in a better way.

A selection can also be made of statements the patients made about nurses. First, in response to the question, 19. "How are the nurses?", the most articulate ones told me:

Patient Aguila: They are very attentive, very kind. They worry about performing their duties in a highly satisfactory way.

Patient Borja: Nurse Arruga treats me badly. The rest are all right.

Patient Dejo: Some are good--- Really, they're all good.

Patient Flores: In Pavilion 4 they mostly treated me well because there was a certain closeness. Things changed when I left there. They treat me badly here, despotically, coldly, unwillingly.

Patient Gálvez: I just know them in passing. Some of them are good.

Patient Justo: They are worthy. They excel in the high level of their behavior. They behave well in their work which is helping the patient or patients, extending to them all kinds of care which is the point of their activities. In sum, I have no complaint about the male nurses or the women nurses.

Patient Lora: There's a young man, B_____, whom they give excessive injections. He's very insolent. The doctors don't notice. They [the nurses] punish him. When a person is lacking in respect or is disobedient, they give him an injection which does harm to his leg and he can't walk for a few days. The one that B_____ had got infected. I get along with almost everybody. They respect me. But they have a certain malice. They need to be ordered more rigorously. They should follow the doctor's orders more strictly. Some of them are student nurses.

Patient Negrín: They obey the doctors' orders.

Patient Ñeco: They're good. I'm a worker here, an active man. I've never had trouble with a nurse.

Patient Salas: They're less attentive. They're short in their attention.

Patient Yáñez: They treat you well, but sometimes they're careless. For example, if you want to talk to the doctor they tell you he doesn't have time.

Two other questions about nurses that elicited some good responses were, 23, "What would you like to receive from them?", and 24, "How should they be? What would be ideal?":

Patient Chocano: 23. That they get closer to us. That at the times when they don't have duties in their office, and when they don't have anything to do, they become our friends, something that would be natural because at home, where people live in common, it becomes indispensable to cultivate friendship. There are no differences within the human species that would stop them, and without prejudice to discipline in the pavilion.

24. They should be more skillful, because the nurse replaces the doctor all the time. Because the nurse lives closer to the patient, he or she can inform the doctor, with greater detail, about his state of improvement, his health, or the process of his illness.

Patient Estrada: 23. What they are giving me, medicines. That's all.

24. Because I don't know anything about medicine, it's hard to answer. I'd like them to be helpful, attentive, and to take care of the patients as the doctor orders.

Patient Flores: 23. What, then? Justice. They are partial. They don't interest me because I've been leading this life for 26 years. The only way I'm going to get out of here is by dying.

24. Justice, which they never practice.

Patient Huerta: 23. Better treatment and medication. With Nurse Arruga, one day I went early to the dormitory where I sleep and she yelled at me. I answered her that I was in a sanatorium not a jail.

24. That they be like other people, that they be correct but not extreme.

Patient Iglesias: 23. More affection.
24. Their good treatment.

Patient Justo: 23. With regard to what? I'd like them to be like the doctors so that they could discharge me already, or let me get out of the Hospital.
24. If they could, to have respect for the patient, to give a little of their best for some patients in the Hospital. For example, that they be less hard. It seems to me that for some patients, who from their illness find themselves with a certain weakness, they ought to be above all magnanimous and good, but they treat them as if they were for the most part already recuperated. It's when they show a certain sadness, a certain melancholy, which becomes quite moving in some cases. The nurses ought to behave their best with patients so that the patients, I imagine, will be cured faster.

Patient Ureta: 23. Service in them. The best thing to receive would be to have them exactly on time, at the correct time.
24. Among themselves they should love each other like companions, so they don't have quarrels or disagreements, so they can live in peace.

Patient Armas: 23. Greater attention, more than they give us, more care, more interest.
24. To carry out what they are taught in the School of Nursing.

A similar series of questions was asked in regard to the attendants. To 26. "How are the attendants?", the fullest responses were:

Patient Aguila: I deal with the attendants very seldom because I'm here in the condition of a convalescent. I've been able to observe that they're educated people. We exchange greetings in a respectful way.

Patient Borja: Some treat me badly. I know them but not their names. They yell at me, nothing more.

Patient Cabral: They're good. I don't see them often. When I ask to be let out [he is a patient with grounds privileges], they open the door for me immediately.

Patient Dejo: They're all good with only one exception, Jiménez. He's not good with me. Several times he left me without tea, without food. When I asked him why he didn't give me tea, he told me that those cups were for the other patients, or that it wasn't the right time to give it. He told me that if I wanted to have tea, I should go home where I could have it at the time I wanted it. He's the only one. All the rest of them are good. Jiménez has treated me with neglect. I've helped them serve breakfast, lunch, tea, dinner many, many times. When I was helping them they treated me well.

Patient Flores: They don't have an alternative. They have to do what their bosses tell them. That's their fate. They can't do anything else.

Patient Huerta: Some of them are--- When you ask them for a little more food, they refuse you. Not all but some of them. . . . I was a paying patient in Pavilion 18. Above all, we had good treatment, with plenty of food. The attendants also had more respect and consideration. They know when you pay. . . . I haven't had any disagreement. I'm only talking about when a person asks for more bread or something more to eat.

Patient Lora: They behave well with me. There's consideration and respect. Some of them treat patients rudely and hit them. Some are lacking in patience.

Patient Márquez: The only one who is gets worried, agitated, is Durán. The rest of them are all right. They obey when you ask for something. . . . Jiménez is the best friend I have here in the pavilion. He took care of me when I came. He gave me advice. He buys me things in stores outside. I don't like Chacón much because he's too young.

Patient Ñeco: They're good. That is, if you don't deal much with them, if you don't have much confidence in them. . . . Disputes occur. I don't speak ill of anyone, but sometimes you can see harsh things when a patient asks for it.

Patient Quintana: They're all bad ones, because they're not good. They don't give good treatment. They fight and use bad language.

Patient Yáñez: Sometimes they don't know how to deal with patients. They treat them harshly. . . . I think Chacón is the nicest one. Some are careless. When shoes need repair or clothing is torn, they don't think about telling the nurse.

Patient Armas: For the most part, they're good. Almost all of them are friends of mine. Some can make me angry. Some don't know their duty. I'd also like to go back to Pavilion 4 because they make me angry. The worst one to me is Hoyos. He always argues with me and that makes me angry. All the rest of them are friends of mine. I have a lot of confidence in them. Some are good; others are all right; and others are very bad. Some of them don't speak respectively, and they use bad language. They call us "crazies" and insult us.

And, finally, to questions, 29, "What would you like to receive from them [the attendants]?" and 30, "How should they be?, what would be ideal?", some patient responses were:

Patient Chocano: 29. From them, nothing.
30. It's necessary to educate them more. That might be done with special courses that would be given them by whomever was competent to do it.

Patient Estrada: 29. What they've always done for me, attention and service.
30. To take care of the patients as the doctor orders, and also to dedicate themselves to other tasks they have to do, like serving food, taking care of some patients who can't take care of their own needs. And---nothing else.

Patient Flores: 29. However they can help. They have to wait on orders from their bosses. If they would want to do something, the doctors would forbid it.
30. That they might be good.

Patient Huerta: 29. Better treatment in the sense of more consideration with food. Because they have a charity pavilion, they think--- There are fights between the attendants and the patients. They don't have consideration. They aren't educated.
30. They should be more agreeable, more human. Although this is a charity pavilion, they ought to have more consideration.

Patient Lora: 29. I'd ask for an improvement in hygiene. When they serve food they seem to be careless. They don't wash the dishes but they fill them again. Some patients are sick and could be contagious. Also, the nurses and attendants don't always wash the things they use for injections. The attendants could clean the bathrooms better.

30. It's necessary to understand the pavilion's needs, to anticipate what the nurses want to help with curing. Their work is routine and simple.

Patient Negrín: 29. Nothing. With other patients, they ought to treat them with a little more consideration. They don't give them clothing or sufficient food. Sometimes they let them fight among themselves. That's bad.

30. Everything is fine, but they ought to be a little more considerate with the patients. Some of them urinate in bed and they hit them. They should realize that they are sick. Aside from that they're good.

Patient Ureta: 29. The service that they give me. I'd like them to let me know if there's any need for my presence.

30. They ought to be respectful, workers, and above all obedient.

Patient Zevallos: 29. I'd like all the personnel here to take me as I am, to forgive me for what I say. If I've done something, there's a reason for it. They'll know, too, how they've found me. My greatest desire is to be good and to change from the life I had before, because we can change ourselves and turn into good people.

30. [This question was not asked.]

Summary and conclusions

Most of the patients see the Hospital passively as a place "to get cured," where care and treatment are given to them. Thus, they want and expect a "cure" or, at least, improvement. At the same time, some of them feel like prisoners, locked up and isolated, confined against their will. They find that, in view of their condition as internal patients, it is hard to get used to it, to adapt to a different kind of existence. One patient feels alone, without anyone's help; another misses his relatives and friends; still others are fearful of a mental hospital, or mental illness, or of being with mental patients: "I never thought I'd be here." "It's a bad dream, a nightmare." "I don't look at the patients, at the horrors." There is fear of the idea of being "crazy," or being called that, as well as fear in the idea that hospitalization could be permanent. Some fear the treatment or the medication. They feel sad, strange, uneasy, in bad humor, vexed, fatigued, with bad thoughts, unable to sleep. They want better or, simply, more food, because it is not like the food at home: it is monotonous, without condiments, and the attendants don't give enough of it, or they refuse to give it. One patient wants to leave in order to forget that he is sick. Another is worried about personal matters, that his relatives will not take care of his things, and another does not want to be a burden on his family. They appear to have the hope for affection at the same time that they experience impenetrable barriers to union with others. And some see the Hospital as a veritable asylum from the poverty, filth, abuse, and horrors of the streets outside, that is, the rest of the world: it is a paradise where one can find peace.

Some of the patients say that it is necessary to be optimistic, or to resign oneself, to be patient, to be at peace, to be responsible, to accustom oneself to the treatment, to reveal everything to the doctor. Others focus more on good behavior: it is necessary to submit to the rules, the discipline; it's necessary to show respect, obey orders, obey personnel. One says that one should not hurt others. Another says that one should behave oneself with the doctors, the nurses, the attendants. They see themselves as helpers, workers who assist by cleaning, serving food, working in the garden, watching out for patients who are sicker than they are, or guarding against escapes. Some say that it is important to be at the doctor's orders, to listen to him, because doctors observe and reveal, and they *know*; while others say that doctors are like jailers, and some of them are violent. Patients want to be the recipients of help, affection, and patience on the part of the personnel. Doctors ought to treat them like good fathers treat their sons. One believes that the doctors are trying to make a person out of him. Nurses ought to be magnanimous with people who are weak; they should not be distant, curt, scolding, careless, or punitive. And attendants should obey their bosses; they should not scream at the patients, hit them, call them bad names, or use bad language with them. Above all, a patient needs to have friends and be friendly with other patients, but not with everyone because some are bothersome and others can inflict damage if one is not careful.

Almost all are agreed in showing their satisfaction with the pavilion which, although it is for charity patients, has a modern construction and contains up to date facilities for sleeping, eating, going to the toilet, and relaxing, while a few miss a more traditional pavilion for poor people.

They recognize the Hospital as the only one for mental illnesses in the country. They say that the pavilion offers rest and health. A minority of patients see it as a jail, a receptacle for "crazies," incurables, and idiots, while others call it a clinic, a hospice, a sanitorium where mental patients are "cured," not an asylum but a hospital that produces healthy people. As some observe, it is a guide for the human mind, or for the development of the human mind.

There is one remaining task for this Chapter, one which relates to a theme that was taken up in Chapter 2. There, in dealing with concepts of mental illness among the different population categories in the Hospital, I noted the differences between the more professional levels, the doctors and nurses, with ones lower in the Hospital hierarchy, the attendants and patients. The discussion ended by pointing to the ideological gap between the elite and the less powerful, suggesting, with regard to the patients, that such a gap was contraindicated in any mental hospital which endeavors to be active therapeutically, because the exclusion of the majority of the population from sharing elite concepts constitutes a dysfunction in the sense that patients might be, thus, cut off from their own therapy.

M. Jones (1962:53) describes the "therapeutic community" as "distinctive among other comparable treatment centers in the way the institutions's total resources, both staff and patients, are self-consciously pooled in furthering treatment. This implies, above all, a change in the usual status of patients. In collaboration with the staff, they now become active participants in the therapy of themselves and other patients and in other aspects of the over-all hospital work--in contrast to their relatively more passive, recipient role in conventional treatment regimes." Then, was Pavilion 20 an antitherapeutic community? Hardly, despite much structural ambivalence, when we examine the data with the goal of looking for possibilities of realizing therapy instead of barriers to it. It is clear that most of the patients, as well as the personnel (see Chapter 3) believe in the Hospital's therapeutic mission. The gap, therefore, is not as wide as one might expect from simply looking at ideological divergences with respect to the etiology of behavioral disorders. If patients know less about the theories of mental illness, it is apparent that many of them are quite knowledgeable about psychotherapy, as we may read into many of their positive testimonies regarding their efforts toward self-acceptance. One admits that his improvement depends on himself; and another affirms that we can change ourselves and turn into good people. These are, indeed, powerful resources for the realization of a more therapeutic hospital.

Appendix I

The list of questions given to the patients is as follows:

1. Name.
2. Age.
3. Place of birth.
4. Diagnosis (provided by the secretary of Pavilion 20).
5. Length of stay in Pavilion 20, in the Hospital.
6. Experience in other pavilions, if any.
7. Experience in other hospitals, if any.
8. Who is your doctor?
9. Do you like him? If not, why?
10. Who is the best doctor? How are the others?
11. How is Pavilion 20 in comparison with other pavilions?
12. Do the doctors give enough time in interviews? In the frequency of interviews?
13. What would you like to receive from them?
14. How would you like the doctors to treat you?
15. What is good in the doctors? What is bad?
16. What would be ideal in the doctor?
17. What kinds of treatment are you getting? (Physical, medications, electro-convulsive, insulin, psychotherapy?)
18. How do you like it (them)? Are you satisfied with the treatment?
19. How are the nurses?
20. How is Pavilion 20 in comparison with other pavilions in regard to the nurses?
21. Which of the nurses do you like most and why?
22. Which do you like least and why?
23. What would you like to receive from the nurses?
24. How should the nurses be? What would be ideal?
25. Do you know any attendants by name? Who are they?
26. How are the attendants?
27. How is Pavilion 20 in comparison with other pavilions in regard to attendants?
28. Which ones do you like most and why? Least and why?
29. What would you like to receive from them?
30. How should be the attendant be? What would be ideal?
31. What contacts do you have with the social workers? With the

psychologists?
32. How are the patients? How do they treat you.
33. Who are your friends? Your best friends?
34. Your best friend?
35. Your dormitory companions?
36. Your dining companions?
37. Your companions in games and sports?
38. If you had leave to go into town for a day, with whom would you like to go?
39. What else do you do with the patients?
40. What things would you like to do?
41. What is the patient's duty?
42. How do you like Pavilion 20 in general?
43. Are you satisfied or not? If not, why?
44. How is Pavilion 20 in relation to other pavilions?
45. How do you like the food?
46. How do you like the clothing? (If he is dressed in Hospital clothing.)
47. How do you like the cleaning?
48. How do you like the rules?
49. Which is your dormitory?
50. Which is the best dormitory and why?
51. Would you like to change dormitories and why?
52. If you had to change dormitories, which would you prefer?
53. What thing ought Pavilion 20 try to do? What is the goal? Why does it exist?
54. Do you think it is doing it? How is it doing it, or how should it do it?
55. What thing ought the Hospital Víctor Larco Herrera try to do? What is the goal? Why does it exist?
56. Do you think it is doing it? How is it doing it, or how should it do it?
57. Does your family come to visit? How many times? Are you satisfied? Would you like to see them more?
58. If you could change something in Pavilion 20, what thing or things would it be?
59. What is mental illness in general? How does it happen. From where does it come?
60. Have your ideas changed after coming here? How? What expectation did you have?
61. What is a hospital like Víctor Larco Herrera?
62. Have your ideas changed after coming here? How? What expectation did you have?
63. What happened to you when you came to the Hospital? To Pavilion 20? How did you feel? What things do you remember more clearly?
64. What things do you consider most important for getting used to it?

65. What were your greatest difficulties?
66. Supposing I were a new patient who had just come, what advice would you give me to get used to it more quickly?

Appendix II

Here a list of the patients interviewed is given, including the following information: fictitious name, date of interview, age, diagnosis, place of birth, time in hospital. The data were kindly furnished by the secretary of Pavilion 20, Señorita Adelinda Horna.

Aguila, 9-29-59, 38, manic-depressive psychosis mania, Lima, 1 year.

Borja, 9-30, 22, anxious reactive depression, South Coast, not indicated, not indicated.

Cabral, 10-2, 42, abnornal psychopathic personality with symptomatic alcoholism, not indicated, 5 months.

Chocano, 10-6, 53, chronic alcoholism with alcoholic psychosis (delerium tremens), North Coast, 2 years.

Dejo, 10-7, 19, manic-depressive psychosis mania, not indicated, 1 year and a half.

Estrada, 10-7, 38, paranoid schizophrenia, not indicated, 5 months.

Flores, 10-9, 51, paranoid schizophrenia paranoia, Callao, 15 years.

Gálvez, 10-9, 32, paranoid schizophrenia, North Highlands, 6 years.

Huerta, 10-13, 36, paranoid schizophrenia, South Coast, 3 months.

Iglesias, 10-14, 29, paranoid schizophrenia, Callao, 1 year.

Justo, 10-27, 33, paranoid schizophrnia, North Coast, 1 year.

Lora, 10-30, 30, catatonic-paranoid schizophrenia, North Coast, 1 year.

Llerena, 11-3, 41, paranoid schizophrenia,North Highlands, 7 years.

Márquez, 11-4, 32, catatonic schizophrenia, South Coast, 3 months.

Negrín, 11-4, 23, paranoid schizophrenia, South Coast, 3 months.

Ñeco, 11-5, 38, paranoid schizophrenia, North Coast, 15 years.

Ortiz, 11-6, 67, manic-depressive psychosis mania, North Coast, 9 years.

Peña, 11-6, 28, catatonic-hebephrenic schizophrenia, South Coast, 2 years.

Quintana, 11-6, 27, catatonic-paranoid schizophrenia, North Highlands, 1 year.

Reyes, 11-10, 22, paranoid schizophrenia, Lima, 5 months.

Salas, 11-10, 60, paranoid schizophrenia, South Highlands, 19 years.

Tapia, 11-10, 37, paranoid schizophrenia, South Coast, 4 years.

Ureta, 11-11, 28, catatonic-paranoid schizophrenia, Lima, 9 months.

Villa, 11-13, 36, paranoid schizophrenia, Lima, 3 months.

Yáñez, 11-13, 21, paranoid schizophrenia, Lima, 9 months.

Zevallos, 11-14, 25, psychomotor epilepsy, Lima, 9 months.

Armas, 12-5, 67, manic-depressive psychosis circular form, North Highlands, 9 years.

Notes

1. The list of questions will be found in Appendix I. A list of the patients interviewed, with some additional information that will not reveal their identities will be found in Appendix II.

2. K. Jones (1991:17-18) makes a similar evaluation of nineteenth century Britain, where "damp and disease-ridden hovels without light or sanitation, the piles of refuse, the filthy and stinking gutters," the people "worse off than wild animals," suggests that those who were admitted to the asylums were relatively fortunate. "Asylums provided better care than prisons or workhouses; patients were fed and clothed, housed in dry wards, looked after, and given medical treatment, and this was more than many of them could hope for in the world outside."

3. All identities of patients and personnel are fictitious. Names have been assigned alphabetically, according to the date of the interview, between September 29 and December 5, 1959. See Appendix II for a list of those patients interviewed.

4. I was to experience the same uncanny feeling thirty years later on a nursing home floor filled with organic brain syndrome cases. I will never forget the first lunch I attended in the day room: about twenty patients divided into groups seated around two large round tables, in stony silence, being fed by nurses' aides, each patient looking straight ahead, nobody talking to anyone else, nobody caring about anything else but the feeding, if that. Suddenly, the realization came to me that I had reached the lowest level of Hades, that there was nowhere to go from there.

5. Problems of social interaction in a psychiatric unit are doubtlessly more complicated than a simple matter of withdrawal. Burnham, Gladstone, and Gibson (1969) suggest that schizophrenia involves a disturbance in object relations. They observe different kinds of patient behavior, including object clinging, object avoidance, substitution of objects, and object redefinition, components of the approach and avoidance characteristic of a "need-fear dilemma."

Chapter 5

Definitions of Social Roles in the Hospital Population: The Family Model

This chapter deals with the definitions made by the several personnel categories of the Hospital of the social roles in the Hospital world, revealed by the interviews I conducted in that population. I asked these people (doctors, nurses, and attendants) to tell me their conceptions of their own obligations and duties, those of the other personnel categories, and those of the patients.[1] They provided a series of images with which a "perceived structure" could be formed, but behind their perceptions I also discovered that I could also construct a "transferred structure" consisting of family images, based on a family model of the Hospital.

Here the concept of transference is applied to the interview materials in order to test such a possibility. I am employing a concept of transference that is broader than what the term usually signifies in psychiatry. Delgado (1989:394-395) defines transference in terms of "the patient's attitude toward the doctor [which] would be the most important factor in the therapeutic process, thanks to which the patient projects unconsciously into the psychoanalyst's person the objects of frustrated love from infancy; and with a kind of polyvalent figurehead, he or she relives and satisfies in a sublimated and delayed way--as one frustrated love from infancy; and with a kind of polyvalent figurehead, he or she relives and satisfies in a sublimated and delayed way--as one who recovers lost time--the sexual desires that were repressed." The idea of transference in the hospital context has been noted by several observers in relation to patients. Sarwer-Foner (1961) speaks of an "institutional transference" in which "the patient unconsciously treats the hospital in the present as though it represented significant past figures in his family," an "affective distortion" which "then becomes an important unconscious factor in his dealings with the hospital." Caudill (1958:157) also uncovers the family model in psychiatric theory which supports the idea that patients are in the position of "children" in the hospital, with the resident physicians and nurses in the positions of "fathers" and "mothers." Cooper (1967:20) notes how, "In the mental hospital, society has, with unerring skill, produced a social structure that in many respects reduplicates the maddening peculiarities of the patient's family. In the mental hospital he finds psychiatrists, administrators, nurses, who are his veritable parents, brothers, and sisters, who play an interpersonal game which only too often resembles in the intricacies of its rules the game he failed at home." Linn (1964:134), on the other hand, views the family model as essential to the formation of a therapeutic milieu in a psychiatric service: "[T]o create a therapeutic milieu in psychoanalytic terms, the ward must be conceived of as a functional unit, and its members as siblings. The staff must be conceived of as another unit, and its members as 'good' parents who provide an opportunity for growth in a rational setting."

What I would like to suggest is that the family model is not simply constructed, or transferred, by patients alone; and, indeed, it also includes a countertransference process that forces us to view it as a collective phenomenon. We confront a situation in which *everyone* participates in this social construction. It is not my intention (or is it?) to view this "transferred structure" as a collective psychopathology (unless it could perhaps be termed a "collective psychopathology of everyday hospital life") but simply as a mental structure created by hospital people, in some cases almost consciously and in others, apparently, unconsciously. Or could it be included in the notion of "closet insanity" constructed by Luske (1990:112-113)? Luske says:

> What is closet insanity and how does it emerge in the first place? Staff are required to construct other people's behavior as symptoms of mental illness. The vast majority of staff believe that psychosis is

> an objective disease entity that causes symptoms in the form of the residents' unusual experiences. Even the minority of staff who resist this model are nonetheless threatened by the possibility of its objective truth. Staff fear that if this model is objectively real, then this same model must apply to their own private experiences since . . . they are often indistinguishable from the public symptoms of the so-called psychotic residents. Thus staff indoctrination into psychiatric ideology . . . can create full-blown closet insanity as self-labeling in accord with its premises.
>
> In looking at the sources of this indoctrination, we see that staff are enmeshed daily in an enormous ideological and institutional apparatus, which, of course, they coauthor. . . . Thus staff's status and role, not to mention economic survival, are thoroughly integrated within this network of social relations as in fact both their producers and products. Given the total hegemony of psychiatric ideology, it is the rare worker able to resist its sway over his/her thought and practice. . . . Is it any wonder, then, that in this atmosphere staff often fear that their own private problems are on the edge of psychosis? As key actors in this "psychiatrization of reality," it could hardly be otherwise. . . . And since staff's daily work reminds them of the bleak consequences that often flow from public displays of unusual experiences, staff hide them in the closet.

In other words, psychiatric personnel tend to expel what is painful from their conscious thought processes. Caudill (1958:13) states:

> [The] question of the binding influence of a social system on unconscious as well as conscious processes needs emphasis and much further exploration, as to date social scientists have not paid much attention to unconscious processes, whether in the study of communities, factories, hospitals, or small groups.

To return, now, to a construction of the family model for a psychiatric hospital: family roles may also be read into Freidson's (1970b:126-127) sociological statements about the principal actors--physicians, nurses, and attendants--within the mental hospital, of whom, he says, the physician

> largely determines what therapeutic efforts are made and, if he does not make all such efforts himself, he orders and supervises the efforts of others. . . . [I]t is the physician's expertise that is his ultimate resource in his interaction with others. As the final arbiter of practice

> in the medical division of labor, sustained by prestige and legal mandate, he has an 'authority' that is independent of administrative authority as such. . . . This leads to hierarchical behavior even in those settings where the philosophy of treatment involves attempts to set up 'democratic' or 'therapeutic communities' which, while nonhierarchical in intent, turn out to be hierarchical in practice. There is no court of appeal from superior training, knowledge, and judgment; technical decisions are not made by vote.

If the physician, who, quite apart from reality, takes on an omnipotent and omniscient character, resembles the ideal "father of the family"--if not the real father or the father who is wished for--, in the sense of exercising male prerogatives on the service, the female nurse (or the male nurse within an unconscious process) can represent the "wife-mother." Freidson (ibid.:126) characterizes "her":

> She is the agent of the supervising physician in carrying out treatment and patient care. In this sense, she represents the professional perspective on the ward. However, insofar as she represents the day-to-day administration of the ward, she is also concerned with patients as a batch . . . . She must, therefore, balance individual physicians' orders for the care of individual patients against the independent demands of the patients as such and against the need to manage an aggregate of cases in an administratively acceptable way. . . . In bargaining with physicians, one of her prime resources lies in her first-hand knowledge and professional evaluation of what goes on in the ward through her continued presence . . . . In bargaining with patients, her prime strength lies in her access to the physician, both in knowing his inside information and in being able to discuss cases with him.

And we can conceptualize the role of attendants as "older siblings" who, in their frequent contacts with the "helpless babies," i.e., the patients, on the service, act as guardians and caretakers, taking directions from the "parents." Freidson (ibid.:124-125) says of them:

> These poorly paid, essentially untrained workers, whose job it is to handle the dirty work of the wards, cannot be expected to hold, much less to exercise, the complex conceptions of treatment espoused by professionals. . . . By virtue of being involved in work on the ward day and night, [they are] in a position to exercise some leverage over the patient, both by physical restraint, and by the age-old evasive

> tactics of the underdog everywhere--"not hearing," "forgetting," and otherwise evading the demands of the more powerful. This certainly gives [them] a position of some influence on any ward. What apparently consolidates and strengthens the aide's position in the state mental hospital, however, is the effective absence from the ward of other workers, combined with circumstances that effectively neutralize patient demands. It seems no accident that these "first-line" workers are powerful precisely in those settings where the patients are stripped of their identity as responsible, adult human beings, and where there is no extensive and continuous participation by professional workers in some regular, effective therapeutic process on or off the wards.

In reality, inside this Hospital, it is not the attendant who is subject to orders (and potentially contradictory ones) from more than one source as much as it is the nurse who is inserted in the structure of the Hospital in a mode that Henry (1954:141) calls "multiple subordination," which is to say that the nurse has more than one superior. Thus, a nurse has to submit not only to the physician's authority but as well to that of the nursing supervisors, which sometimes presents problems in the functioning of the pavilions and the Hospital. Moreover, the nurses, in spite of their struggles to see themselves as professional persons, are effectively employees, as Rubenstein and Lasswell (1966:61) point out, and thus do not expect to "dominate or contribute to a field of knowledge," but experience "the context of the hospital and its activities with relatively little intellectualization." While the attendants are also subject to the authority of the nursing supervisors, they are given their orders by the nurses in the pavilions. They have many fewer contacts with the physicians whose greater interests are focused on the patients. Salisbury (1962:50) observes that they are present on the service but ignored by the physicians who only notice those who can give them the information they need. Although they have constant and intensive contact with the patients, according to Straus, et al. (1963:157), "they are considered quite secondary to the therapeutic process."

Clearly, the family model in the Lima Hospital was "contaminated" by the conditions under which it existed, particularly the political control exerted by the Public Charity Society of Lima through the Hospital's administrator who favored the administration and refused to give the psychiatric personnel the resources they badly needed for their services. But general poverty ruled not only in the Hospital but in the city of Lima and in the national context. Stipends and wages were low, and almost everyone had to look for additional sources of income. Not only did the physicians have to put together a personal income from different sources, but the nurses, too, worked their shifts in the Hospital and often second shifts in other hospitals or in the homes of private patients. The attendants also worked at other jobs; and many of them expected to change their work, preferably to occupations where they could pursue their own interests as petty tradespersons. It is quite apparent that few if any of the Hospital personnel were focused exclusively on their lives and social relations within the Hospital. In no way were they actually like members of a family. This was the context in which I sought the views of the several categories of Hospital personnel on their Hospital roles.

The Psychiatrists

To begin presentation of the data, let us examine the role conceptions of the psychiatrists as seen by both themselves and paramedical personnel. I asked twelve subjects, all males, "What is the doctor's duty?," and received these responses:

> Dr. Alba[2]: The treatment of his patients.
>
> Dr. Bueno: He has to be in touch with the evaluation of each patient, if the latter has received the treatment prescribed or has been forgotten, so that he can recover from those problems, because the health of the patient comes above everything else. And the doctor has to think about each one of his patients on the service, because that's his duty.
>
> Dr. Caso: It would be to carry out the mission which belongs to him in the distribution of work, to take care of urgent situations, and to collaborate with the other doctors in the work they are called on to do.
>
> Dr. Chávez: You have to agree with psychiatric knowledge in order to answer the question. Empirically, I can tell you, it's the interview. You have to be a doctor who is in touch with all the different manifestations a mental patient can present.
>
> Dr. Díaz: The doctor has to restore patients to the group, to

society. He has to do everything possible. If it's not possible, he has to put them in the kind of condition where they can do a bit of work, where they feel useful.

Dr. Espinoza: In the first place, he must dedicate himself completely to the patients with a constructive purpose. It's most important that they receive something, at least a social remission, without ignorning the other patients. Then he has to carry on daily conversations with them. They're isolated and they need to be entertained in their intellectual lives. And he has to give direction to the personnel so that they can take better care of psychiatric patients.

Dr. Fernández: The doctor has to see to the good care of patients, that they receive good treatment from everybody, so that the personnel want patients to be considered as human beings and not as cases.

Dr. Gómez: He has to give immediate attention to the patient, if he needs something, and give physical treatment if it is necessary.

Dr. Herrera: To do everthing in my power to cure and rehabilitate curable patients. In the case of chronic patients, to make it so that during their stay in the Hospital they are maintained on human levels. It's understood that duty is unavoidable in the clinical aspect, but in this Hospital it's also unavoidable sometimes to act on extra-clinical terrain.

Dr. Ibarra: Being as efficient and responsible in his work as possible.

Dr. Jara: To care for patients with reassurance, understanding, and doing research.

Dr. López: To find the cure and in any case the well being of the patient and his family, for which he has to study each case carefully and keep himself on a plan of constant training for study and research.

The 13 nurses, 7 men and 6 women,[3] I interviewed gave me a different and complementary series of responses to the questions, "How are the doctors? How do they treat you?," "How should the doctor be?," and "What is the doctor's principal duty?":

Nurse Arruga [only to the first two questions]: They're all more or less good. I can't complain about any of the doctors I know in the Hospital. They treat me well.

A doctor should behave like a professional, be responsible, be a gentleman, and have love for his work.

Nurse Bustos: The new doctors, the boys, are more understanding. They treat you like a collaborator. The older medical personnel don't treat us very well. They give orders and you are required to obey. They abuse nurses physically, Dr. Lleras, for example. He hasn't learned. . . . All the student nurses are afraid of him. It's fear more than respect.

He should work with the nurse in mutual accord creating, as you say, a therapeutic atmosphere.

It would be his professional ethics.

Nurse Cruz: They're good. There are all kinds. Here they treat us very well, but in other places other doctors have a very different manner where they believe they are the only ones and that the nurse is on a different level. There are exceptions in all hospitals, even this one. There are doctors who don't have manners.

The doctor should tell the nurse how he ought to be, because the nurse isn't a person who's been prepared. He's done his primary and secondary studies and as such he's a person that can relate to him. As human beings we all have the right to be treated as such.

He ought to be for his patient as far as the recovery of both physical and mental health goes, and confront the patient with the way he ought to be. He should concentrate on the truth and not tell him, "All right, all right, such and such is going to happen." We have the case of a disturbed patient, and the doctor says, "Good, let's give him such and such a treatment," and then he leaves and the matter falls into the nurse's hands. And then the patient blames the nurse for not carrying out what the doctor had ordered. That's something that happens generally.

Nurse Chivas: They're good. They have a lot of confidence in their nurses, and the nurses have to cooperate with them. The nurse is the doctor's right arm. You have to know how to deal with them. The atmosphere has a great deal of influence on the personality of the doctor and of the nurse. It's like a mirror in which they see themselves. If you don't have a strong personality, you can suffer from the same disturbances. It's easy to lose your balance. I've seen many cases of personnel who've got sick. If you don't know how to behave, you can get sick. That's the great disadvantage that this work has. Some doctors also suffer. The atmosphere has a lot of influence on the doctors, the nurses, and the attendants.

It depends. Each person has formed his personality. You have to know how to behave. You can't be temperamental. This atmosphere is a bad one.

The doctor directs the treatment and the nurse is the one who executes it. The doctor gives orders and the nurse carries them out. The doctor gives the treatment and we follow his orders.

Nurse Delgado: They're good, pleasant, and kind. There exists a partnership between the doctor and the nurse.

There's a lot of understanding between the doctor and the nurse.

He should be constantly concerned about his patients, so that they don't miss anything in their treatment, and he should also watch for the slow recuperation of his patients and see that everybody cooperates.

Nurse Esquivel [only to the second and third questions]: He ought to be quite punctual in his visits. Dealing with the patient is his business. The ideal would be to have his cooperation with the nurse in the many aspects of the work.

That's for the doctor to answer. I've said punctuality and frequency.

Nurse Frías [only to the second and third questions]: The doctor ought to be a serious man who makes himself respected by all the personnel. He should have his orders for the patients carried out well. He should have initiative to improve the pavilion. Without this support a nurse can't do anything

I've already said he has to see to the well being of his patients. Some of them ask for a change in nurses because they don't like them. He has to carry out all his obligations.

Nurse Godoy [only to the second and third questions]: He should watch the patients and look for their cure. He should watch treatment continually so that he can know how the patient is progressing. He should dedicate himself to rounds, to conversing with them. He should talk with each one for a few minutes every day. Some doctors don't know the patients. That's intolerable.

He should be concerned about his patients and see that they don't go without their medicine.

Nurse Hurtado: They're good. I can't complain about any of them.
He ought to be interested at all times in the patient's recuperation.
He should study conscientiously the different cases he sees and carry out treatments.

Nurse Iglesias: They're my superiors. They treat me well.
He ought to make his rounds, indicate treatment for them. He should have understanding.
He should direct the nurse and check on what he ordered the day before.

Nurse Justo: You have to know how to adapt yourself to each one of them.
He should carry out his duty strictly.
He should carry out his obligations.

Nurse Lozada: They are very friendly.
He has to give attention to the patient.
He should come to the Hospital every day and watch the patients.

Nurse Llosa: We have a rational hierarchy. There should exist pleasantness and understanding.
He should carry out his duties.
He should carry out his profession with integrity.

A sample of 17 attendants, 13 men and 4 women,[4] gave me still another perspective--one radically different in content--with their responses to the questions, "How are the doctors? How do they treat you?" and "How should the doctor be?":

Attendant Alfaro: All right. They're good. Nothing has happened with us yet. They act all right.
When the doctor calls us, we have to be at his orders quickly. We have to know what they're asking us and how to satisfy them.

Attendant Bravo: All the doctors treat me well.
A doctor has to look after the pavilion's progress. That includes everything, the patients, the personnel, everything we do.

Attendant Costa: They treat us well.
I can't answer. They should be persons who get along well with all the personnel and the patients.

Attendant Chacón: They all treat us well.
I don't know.

Attendant Durán: They're good, pleasant. They treat me well.
He ought to be generous for humanity.

Attendant Estrada: They're very good. I'm always asking them for favors. When my son was sick they took care of him. All the doctors here are very fine.

They should conduct themselves so as to get to know the attendant. In other pavilions if you say to the doctor, "Please give me a pill because I'm not feeling well," he refuses; but here they give it to you. They're all the same. I can ask a favor of any of them and they do it.

Attendant Fuentes: They're good. They treat us with good manners.

The doctor ought to be generous with the attendants. He ought to know how to be good to them.

Attendant García: They go on rounds, they look after the patients, they see that they're clean.

They should show their kindness and their trust in the inferior, as much toward the patients as toward the attendants. They should tell you how things are, how the patients are behaving.

Attendant Hoyos: They're good. They treat me well.
They should treat us well and be friendly.

Attendant Ibáñez: I can't tell you anything because I don't know them. They treat me well.

The doctor should be good and do favors for the attendants. They ought to look at the attendants when they get sick. They ought to give them prescriptions and examinations.

Attendant Jiménez: They're very good. Up to now they're treated me well.

As a doctor he has the right to make known all the knowledge that an attendant doesn't know.

Attendant León: They are good people, helpful. If you ask them for a favor they help you. A few days ago I asked Dr. Alba for a prescription and he gave it to me. He gave me a box of medicine, too.

He ought to be up to date with the patients and give them the right treatment that they deserve. The doctors are in charge of the patients' health, better to say the whole world's health.

Attendant Llona: They have good characters. They treat us with consideration.

He ought to give all his attention to his patients so as to be more important and have a larger clientele.

Attendant Meza: Most of them are good in the way they treat you, the way they order something urgent.

The doctor has to be good. He should treat a person for anything, and give orders calmly and peacefully.

Attendant Nores: They are good, easy to get along with.

They should be easy to get along with, not arrogant. Sometimes when a person greets them, they reject him. That could be because they're very busy.

Attendant Ortiz: They're good. . . . They treat us very well. It's the same in other pavilions. Since we deal with them very seldom we don't have any complaints.

He should have character, know how to deal with personnel.

Attendant Paredes: They're good. They treat me well.

He should be good and treat personnel well.

The Nurses

Let us now examine the nurse's role from the points of view of the different categories of Hospital personnel. The same group of nurses, in response to two questions, "What importance has the nurse in the Hospital?" and "What is the nurse's greatest duty?," revealed aspects of their self-concept:

Nurse Arruga [only to the first question]: Without the nurse, things wouldn't happen in the Hospital. She has to make things get done, over and over, especially in mental hospitals. Without it the cleaning wouldn't get done and the negative patients wouldn't eat.

Nurse Bustos: He's the one who distributes work to all the attendants. He shows them the work, as well as working himself.

Collaborating with the doctor

Nurse Cruz: He collaborates with the doctors because, otherwise, with whom would the doctor work. Alone? The doctor doesn't remain for long.

The nurse has to look after the patients' care, and make sure that nothing happens with them, that they don't harm each other, everything in relation to their persons. He has to teach them certain principles that they need, like the form of living they ought to follow when they're discharged.

Nurse Chivas: I think he is indispensable, like a father at home. He's the treatment base because he informs the doctor about his observation of the patient all day long.

He has to help the patient in every possible way with his problems and health. You have to resolve a variety of problems here, from food and clothing to treatment.

Nurse Delgado: She's an indispensable person for the service, as much for the doctors as for the patients, for the administration of the pavilion.

You have to try to get the patient to cooperate with you, and you should make yourself liked and respected so that the patient does everything you tell him to do with affection.

Nurse Esquivel [only to the second question]: He has to lend himself wholly to the greatest assistance of the patients.

Nurse Frías [only to the second question]: She should strictly carry out the doctors' orders for treatment.

Nurse Godoy [only to the first question]: Her importance in relation to patients is clear. She's the doctor's right hand. The doctors only come for a few minutes and the nurse tells them how the patients are.

Nurse Hurtado: Of course he's important. The role is so important that without nursing there wouldn't be medicine.

In the first place, he has to see to good care and the carrying out of all doctors' orders. Then he has to watch the discipline that should exist in the pavilion.

Nurse Iglesias: She's responsible for the service to which they send her, and she executes what the doctors prescribe.

She has to carry out strictly orders by the doctors of the service.

Nurse Justo: She's important in every way within her duties and obligations.

She has to carry out her duty within her schedule.

Nurse Lozada: The importance is in the responsibility he has in his functions.

He should come to work every day and be watchful with the patients.

Nurse Llosa: The nurse is the doctor's first assistant.

He has to practice his profession with integrity.

In contrast, the doctors responded to the question, "What is the nurse's duty?," as follows:

Dr. Alba: To collaborate with the doctor in the application of care and treatment for the patients.

Dr. Bueno: To carry out the doctor's orders, mend the holes, consult with the doctor about the problems he finds, not to create problems among the attendants or the nurses, and, last of all, with anybody. Nurses should slip softly and peacefully around the pavilion carrying out their duties. They shouldn't arrive late or leave the pavilion they're assigned to during working hours, except in cases of real emergency.

Dr. Caso: It's also something similar to the doctor, but within their functions. One duty is insulin therapy, and they ought to carry that out in the best way possible. The role relates to their work in giving care to the patient, the carrying out of doctors' orders. One characteristic is that nurses also take care of patients, but they do it according to our directions, according to the guides we give them. They shouldn't get distracted by other things.

Dr. Chávez: There are two things: first, carrying out what has been ordered for treatment on that day; second, explaining or reporting on everything that happens with the patients, that can be expressed in their language. A nurse should be alert to anything new that can come up among the patients, and let others know about it immediately.

Dr. Díaz: I think there ought to be a team of persons, all working for themselves and all following the same goal, with the same principles and ends. That way, patients can be useful if they can't go back to their groups. This would be a prophylactic labor. Then the public would have more confidence. I think that people are very mistrustful and keep on thinking of patients in the same way as before: that they are lost.

Dr. Espinoza: To reduce or avoid conflicts among the patients, trying always to isolate the most aggressive ones. Then a nurse ought to see to it that the ones with homosexual tendencies are present and counted, and inform the medical personnel about this. Also, to have an appreciation of the psychic state that each patient finds himself in and the treatment he is receiving. Like that, the nurse can face any situation with exact information.

Dr. Fernández: To carry out doctors' orders, report on the patients' state so as to come upon symptoms and any intent of aggression or abnormal conduct that would be harmful to themselves or to the pavilion. Cordial treatment of patients is necessary.

Dr. Gómez: In the first place, vigilance and being alert to communicate anything new to the doctor.

Dr. Herrera: The nurse should be concerned with aspects relating to the patient's comfort during his stay in the Hospital, and with following orders that the doctor gives regarding the treatment that is to be followed in each case.

Dr. Ibarra: Open collaboration with the doctor, carrying out orders, spontaneity, and responsibility.

Dr. Jara: Collaboration with the doctor in treating the patients.

Dr. López: Helping the doctor in his labors and making the patient's existence more bearable, and giving all the support and help possible to the relatives.

The nurse's role as viewed by the attendants was approached by means of three questions, "How are the nurses? How do they treat you?," "How should a nurse be?," and "Which of the nurses do you like most? Least?":

Attendant Alfaro: They're good people, very kind. There still hasn't been anything to the contrary.

The first thing is to be a little strict. Sometimes they're a little short, and other times they're better. We have to be at their orders.

For me it's the same as any job. If you behave yourself there's no problem. In other pavilions it's something else.

Attendant Bravo [only to the first two questions]: Up to now I don't have any complaint about them.

The nurse also has to see to it that the service responds to the sacrifice she's making.

Attendant Costa: The nurses' treatment of the attendants is good.

A nurse should be a good person and have good treatment for all the attendants and patients.

Señorita Arruga has a good way of working. I'm not intimate or friendly with any of them.

Attendant Chacón: They treat me well.

A nurse should be in mutual accord with the attendant.

Señorita Arruga is more serious and better. She doesn't refuse anything on the service that you ask her for. I like Señora Frías less because of the way she treats you.

Attendant Durán: They are also good, kind, attentive. They treat me affectionately.

They should work pleasantly with the attendants in order to serve their patients.

They're the same for me.

Attendant Estrada [only to the first two questions]: Señora Frías is very good. Sometimes Señorita Arruga scolds an attendant. Señor Muelle is a bit excitable. He doesn't know how to take charge of the pavilion. Yesterday he had us going upstairs and downstairs with cots, and from dormitory to dormitory. Señor Hurtado is a nice person, also Señor Bustos. Señor Cruz is something of an informer. Ch_____ [a patient] was fighting with [Attendant] Chacón and Señor Cruz told the doctor. All the attendants think he's an informer.

A nurse has to see if the attendant is a worker, and if not to change him.

Attendant Fuentes: For me they're all good. They treat me in a good way.

They ought to know how to treat an attendant.

There are very few nurses here. For me, I think all of them are good. I dislike none of them. They're all the same.

Attendant Garcia: In that there are some who act all right and others are a little bad.

That should be the aim with the attendants, acting all right. Sometimes they're a little hard to understand. They don't see their own faults. They shove blame on the attendants.

I've worked for a long time with Nurses Bustos and Cruz. They're good people. They act quite all right. I've been with the others just for short times.

Attendant Hoyos: They get along well with me and with my companions.

They ought to have a way of ordering an attendant, because there are many of them who treat us as if we weren't persons. They treat us very badly. A comrade who lives nearby got sick and asked me to let them know that he couldn't come to work. That nurse asked me why he sent the message, because he had to be seen [i.e., in person], and that he should get well. Well, I didn't tell him to get sick! That happened in Pavilion [n] when I went there to tell Nurse Esquivel. He's the only one who's treated me like that. All my companions know him for his bad treatment of attendants.

I like Señora Frías the most, because any favor I ask her for, like changing shifts, she does for me. I like them all. I chose her because I like her, because she's kinder.

Attendant Ibáñez: They're good. They treat us well here.

They should be easy to get along with and know how to treat an attendant. Then he will respect them.

Señorita Frías because she's easy to get along with. She knows how to deal with a person and she makes no distinctions. She treats everybody the same. I like Señor Muelle less, maybe because I don't know him well. He's new here.

Attendant Jiménez: They're almost all good. Almost all of them are the same. They all treat attendants the same.

It would be that as a nurse he ought to understand an attendant. He should know all the circumstances of an attendant, what he needs, and he also ought to give explanations of how an attendant should treat the patients, especially when they are in a risky treatment.

I like Señora Frías and Señor Bustos because they get along easily with the personnel and they know how to behave well as nurses with the attendants. Señor Muelle is new and I like him less, mainly because as a nurse he doesn't let a person get to know him, and he's not capable of giving orders to an attendant about doing his tasks. They say in Pavilion [n] that he likes working with everything in disorder. It would be his character, his way of doing things.

Attendant León: For me they all give the same treatment. They're all easy to get along with. They know how to give orders. It's the same in their way of dealing with a person.

They should get along well with the attendant and treat him well, respect him, so that attendants will act with good will and respect them on their part.

Because I'm used to it, I'd rather deal with Señora Frías. It's because she's been here a long time. She's quite good and easy to get along with. But they're all the same. I can't say that I like one more and another less. I obey all of them when they give me orders.

Attendant Llona: They're good but they also have moments when they speak to us in a loud voice, maybe with anger. They get along well with the patients. In case some patient creates some disorder, the nurse is charged with giving him some injection so he will be tranquilized, or otherwise another injection so he'll lose the use of his leg, so he won't escape. They scold because sometimes a person comes to work late, and sometimes when we let a lucid patient go into town without telling them, and other times when we don't have the patients in order, when their clothes are dirty or their overalls are wet. That's why the nurse gets angry.

The nurse on the service ought to behave with the attendants as if they were her true friends. She should treat them well, and the same, too, with the patients.

By her character, and in everything, I like Señorita Arruga the most, for the way she orders an attendant to do his jobs. I like Señor Muelle the least because when a person is doing the cleaning in his section he makes him go somewhere else with a message. It shouldn't be like that. He ought to wait for a person to finish something before he starts him on something new.

Attendant Meza: They're good. They treat me well.

They should get along well with the attendants and the patients. That way a person can work in peace.

There are three nurses who are all right because they treat us and the patients with kindness, with kindness and calmness.

Attendant Nores: Some are condescending and others don't have good ways of treating people. They are despots. Sometimes they think that everybody feels the same way. Some of them are educated and know how to deal with people.

A nurse should be a little less selfish and be a little easier to get along with. Some have to keep calling our attention to unimportant things, sometimes for no good reason.

There's a lot of difference between the older ones and the young ones. They can both be selfish. There was one time I was in *laborterapia* [labor therapy[5]] by one's orders and another ordered me out of there. Well, one always has to obey. Some of them tell you why and others don't give any explanation at all. Some are demanding and they call a person ill-bred or unmannerly. That happens when you protest or show that something is not so.

Attendant Ortiz [only to the two first questions]: They are very good. The head of Pavilion [n] is Señorita Rosa Navarro. Now she's on vacation and her second is in charge.

To be respected, a nurse ought to have character. Everything good has to have its bad side, but they're all very good.

Attendant Paredes [only to the first two questions]: The head nurse is very good.

She should be good with the personnel, of course. She should treat them well. She shouldn't tell them how to do something when they're doing it, because they already know how.

The Attendants

The attendants responded to the questions, "What importance does the job of attendant or laborer have in the Hospital?" and "What is the main duty of the attendant?" While only the last three attendants interviewed were asked the second question, the data are sufficient to allow us to complete a picture of the attendants' conception of their own role:

Attendant Alfaro: We are laborers and others are public employees. We aren't public employees but workers. That's given in the Social Security files.

Attendant Bravo: The attendant has a lot of importance, first of all in looking after the patients, taking care of them. The attendants are a great aid to the nurses. It's a help for them. What would they do without the attendants?

Attendant Costa: He has the obligation of looking after the patients and taking care of them.

Attendant Chacón: It's important that he's present to take care of the patients because sometimes they fight. There are times when they could kill each other.

Attendant Durán: Yes, it's important in the sense of helping in treatments that are given to the patients on orders from the nurses or the doctors.

Attendant Estrada: An attendant watches the patients. The importance is in doing their cleaning.

Attendant Fuentes: Of course it's important because the attendant is always called on to do the cleaning.

Attendant García: An attendant has to carry out his work, fulfill his obligation, cooperate.

Attendant Hoyos: Yes, he's important because he lends his services.

Attendant Ibáñez: It's important because the obligation consists of having the service clean and everything in its place.

Attendant Jiménez: We have to obey superiors' orders. It's important because that's the way you show your boss that you can carry out the job you've been hired to do by yourself, without the bosses needing to be watching you.

Attendant León: Of course, it's important. The importance is that we're often here because work outside is inconvenient.

Attendant Llona: Yes, it's very important in the first place to make up the service in the section where the nurse sends you. You have to do the cleaning and watch the patients, and do what the nurse orders.

Attendant Meza: Without attendants there'd be a lot of fights among the patients, so it's the control a person has in being together with them all the time.

Attendant Nores: Important? I don't think so. But it's always necessary that personnel be here. If there weren't personnel the patients would do what they wanted, hitting each other and fighting.

The attendant has to do what the boss orders. She always has to respect the boss and all superiors, and obey orders.

Attendant Ortiz: Yes, it's important for the patients. We have the responsibility of taking care of them. If something happens, they suspend us. If they escape and return home, they suspend us for two or three days.

You have to watch the patients and see that they're not away from where they ought to be. The people can't clean up themselves.

Attendant Paredes: Well, it's done. Yes, it's important to know about.

The attendant has to do her duties, what's assigned to her.

The doctors responded to the question, "What is the attendant's duty?," as follows:

Dr. Alba: It's also care of patients.

Dr. Bueno: It's to be good with the patient, take care of his food, the cleaning of the service, and behave well with them. If there's some serious emergency, he should ask the head nurse to talk to the doctor about solving problems. The attendant ought to be at work on time.

Dr. Caso: It's similar to the doctor's duty, and that of the nurse. He has to perform his role: non-medical work. It's work in cleaning or door-keeping, things like that. Attendants should cooperate with the doctors. It would be a common thing. But attendants have to deal with the patients in doing their work, so that they participate in therapy in a certain way.

Dr. Chávez: In the first place, working, that is, cooperating with the nurse in everything that has to do with the care of patients that doesn't have direct relation to medical matters. Apart from that, he can do everything.

Dr. Díaz: Cooperate in the same way. He should understand patients more. The attendant isn't educated. He insults them, devalues them, and thinks they are crazy. Attendants are uncultured people. It's the lack of preparation.

Dr. Espinoza: The attendant is dedicated to administrative work. He gives all kinds of information to the ones who need it. There's no definite function. Attendants help with what the service asks them for.

Dr. Fernández: He carries out the orders of his immediate superiors. He reports immediately to the nurses on whatever abnormality he observes in direct dealings with the patients, whom in turn he has to help in everything they need: stimulating the apathetic ones, separating the ones who are disturbing the group, and putting to work the patients who are in condition to work.

Dr. Gómez: His duty is strictly vigilance.

Dr. Herrera: Specialized personnel practically don't exist in the pavilion. The attendant's duty is currently limited to cleaning tasks. The exceptions to this rule, like the job of secretary and the work of the head of the *laborterapia* shop, are filled by older attendants who perform these more specialized kinds of work for the same wages.

Dr. Ibarra: Cooperate with the doctor and nurses in the management of patients. They have to be disciplined and attentive in their behavior.

Dr. Jara [did not answer the question].

Dr. López: Satisfy as far as possible the needs of the patient, helping the nurse and, like her, observing, taking care of, and assisting the patient and his family.

The nurses responded to four questions about the attendants, "How are the attendants?," "How should the attendant be?," "Which of the attendants do you like most? Less?," and "What is the attendant's main duty?":

Nurse Arruga [only to the first three questions]: Some are good but others are a little careless. You always have to watch them, but basically they're good.

It would be if you give them an order, some know their jobs and it isn't necessary to reprimand them. An attendant ought to know how to carry out his obligations.

Estrada is a good worker. Costa is a boy but he's respectful. Ibáñez is also a worker, like García and Estrada. The others aren't. Really, I don't dislike anyone. I'm indifferent.

Nurse Bustos: In this pavilion they act all right. They cooperate well in all the orders a nurse gives.

They need to know how to treat patients. They should receive an education for treating mental patients. They should be educated and responsible.

I like the one who works with me [in insulin shock therapy], García, and the boy Jiménez. They are the ones who work best. I deal very little with the others.

To be responsible.

Nurse Cruz: The ones here are good.

An attendant should be prepared. He should know about life because, otherwise, a nurse can be antagonistic toward them. A nurse shouldn't allow one to disobey and not respond to orders. A person who doesn't obey doesn't know his duties. To avoid all that, an attendant should be a person who is capable of accepting advice, explanations, objections, because otherwise they can believe that you're bad, that you like to bother them and be a problem for them.

He should be scrupulous with the patient and with the rest of the professional personnel.

For me they're all the same. They always follow orders. They're always agreeable. I like it least when I work with ones who don't cooperate. They're all good here. There aren't any bad ones. They're always willing.

Nurse Chivas [only to the first two and the last questions]: It's necessary to prepare them from the time they start work in a service, and their work then depends on this preparation.

They should always have instruction so as to be able to take care of patients, because a person always needs to know ways to get along with them and lead them.

They take care of the domestic part. They clean, bring food, and take care of the patients. This is their obligation.

Nurse Delgado [only to the first two and the last questions]: They're all obedient, respectful, and workers.

She should be respectful to her superiors and there should be understanding with everybody so that everybody will help and the service will be in good condition.

That the patient has all the conveniences, like, for example, that she has her dormitories clean and has her equipment in order.

Nurse Esquivel [only to the second and last questions]: He should be cooperative, intelligent, and efficient with all the orders he receives from the nurse.

Cooperation, not only broad but intelligent. Some are obtuse and we have trouble with them.

Nurse Frías: They're good but they always have to be watched because otherwise they don't do what they're supposed to.

Respectful with their superiors. They should do what they're supposed to do and not wait for the nurse to be on top of them. Obedience.

They're all the same. I'm indifferent.

It's being obedient. He should be pleasant with the patients and get along with them.

Nurse Godoy [only to the first two and last questions]: There are all kinds, some of them very understanding and there are other bad ones who even hit them. You always have to watch them. Some are lazy and need to be watched. There are others who are responsible. Men are more responsible than women. The worst male attendant is better than a woman attendant. Some women don't do what they're supposed to do, even when you explain it to them very carefully.

An attendant should understand the patient. Some believe that the patients are insulting them. There are patients who are hallucinating. Once there was an attendant who complained that a patient was insulting her. They get angry, or even more disturbed that the patients, and this bothers the patients. Some attendants understand and are more careful.

The attendant ought always to carry out what has been ordered. She ought to fulfill her obligations.

Nurse Hurtado [only to the first two and last questions]: Here the attendants are almost the nurse's immediate helpers.

They ought to have a short course of preparation for the good treatment of the patient.

An attendant should look out for the general care of the patient.

Nurse Iglesias [only to the first two and last questions]: Some are workers but others are a little slack.

He should do domestic service and watch out that the patients who go into the patio are all right.

Perform service.

Nurse Justo [only to the first two and last questions]: They need preparation.

He should carry out his obligations and obey the rules.

Carry out obligations.

Nurse Lozada [only to the first two and last questions]: They are people without responsibility.

Cleaning the pavilions and watching the patients.

Obey the nurses' orders.

Nurse Llosa [only to the first two and last questions]: They're insufficient and in some cases irresponsible because of their lack of preparation. A school should exist.

Their duty is respect for the patient, for his state and relation to the personnel.

Carry out obligations.

The Patients[6]

The doctors were asked, "What is the patient's duty?," and responded as follows:

Dr. Alba: It depends on the type of patient. It's accepting the efforts of the doctors to help him.

Dr. Bueno: To cooperate with the doctor, accepting the therapeutic measures that are ordered, communicating what he feels and everything that happens in relation to his person. Also, to get along with the nurses and attendants.

Dr. Caso: In the first place, most of the patients don't think they are patients. Apart from this their duty is to cooperate in the way they can. But a patient has his limitations from the illness itself. One of the symptoms can be non-cooperation, and so one can't ask for cooperation as their duty because they're sincere.

Dr. Chávez: This is a function of the critical capacity of the patient, because the mental patient receives more than he can give. He has to be taken care of more than carry out or have duties.

Dr. Díaz: There are so many types that it's a difficult question. I don't think that they ought to have a duty, but rather a great spirit of collaboration.

Dr. Espinoza: His first duty is to obey all the orders given by the doctor. Then the patient himself has the duty of attending on the service punctually when he's been granted leave. And giving reports, for example, on the names of his relatives, so that they can be contacted. That's all.

Dr. Fernández: To follow the establishment's discipline, receive the treatments that are ordered, help each other with a great sense of responsibility, and join in the work of the Hospital.

Dr. Gómez: He should cooperate in his treatment. Even in this pavilion there's always treatment, even if it's limited.

Dr. Herrera: The patient's duty is, within his limitations, to follow the orders of the attending physician and the nurse. The question is debatable in itself, because the performance of duties can't be demanded in those cases where the patient doesn't have a sense of responsibility.

Dr. Ibarra: To make an effort to carry out medical directions, to try to understand his special condition as a sick person, and to help with his cooperation in medical tasks and those of the auxilliary personnel.

Dr. Jara: To submit to treatment with complete trust and to participate actively in the Hospital's progress by taking part in different activities that are compatible with the type and degree of his illness.

Dr. López: To have trust in the doctor, follow his orders, and help in every way that is possible for him toward the progress of our medical knowledge, provided this has no negative effect on his health and comfort.

The nurses also responded to the same question, "What is the patient's main duty?":

Nurse Arruga: To be respectful and cooperate in his treatment. Also, it depends on the condition of each patient and his culture. Is he respectful? You can't make a comparison of D_____ with S_____. Their manners are different. The two cooperate: they take their pills. D_____ is an educated man and can't be rude. But if S_____ is rude, it's his culture, his manner.

Nurse Bustos: Allow himself to be treated.

Nurse Cruz: Follow orders, both in medical and in nursing care. As patients they have to take orders for their improvement or cure, and submit to the Hospital's rules.

Nurse Chivas: Respect the personnel. All the patients have to respect the white coat when they see it. White clothing is for doctors and nurses. The patient has to obey and cooperate.

Nurse Delgado: Cooperate in his treatment and in his recuperation.

Nurse Esquivel: The question isn't clear. The patient has to do what is arranged for him. He has to eat and go to bed at set times. He has to be at the nurse's orders for all the circumstances that can occur. You can't ask a seriously ill patient to have an obligation or a duty.

Nurse Frías: To be reachable or to be obedient for his treatment.

Nurse Godoy: To have respect for the orders of the doctor and the nurse. To collaborate in his treatment. Some reject that and don't even want to take their medication. There are patients who hide their pills under their tongues. The family has to pay for them, and medications are expensive. The patient has to adapt to circumstances. One patient here has spent twenty years in her room. She can't speak to the other patients but feels superior. She is from Arequipa and only wants to speak to the doctors and nurses. For her, the others are crazy.

Nurse Hurtado: He should carry out all the doctor's orders obediently. Then he has to observe the discipline that should exist in the pavilion.

Nurse Iglesias: To obey, follow the rules that exist in the pavilion.

Nurse Justo: To carry out the doctor's orders.

Nurse Lozada: To be respectful and carry out orders given by the professionals.

Nurse Llosa: Obedience and knowing how to adapt to the service.

The same question was given to the attendants, who responded as follows:

Attendant Alfaro: Above all, he has to be at the attendant's orders. To be obedient and not be aggressive. The attendant can't do them favors if they misbehave. If they behave themselves, the attendant has the right to take good care of them, if they're grateful.

Attendant Bravo: They don't have duties. Only the lucid ones have duties. Only they can.

Attendant Costa: It's getting along with the attendants.

Attendant Chacón: It's obeying the attendants, and the nurse.

Attendant Durán: They should obey the attendants.

Attendant Estrada: To look to the attendant, so as not to hit another patient. Some of them are very good. They help.

Attendant Fuentes: They don't have responsibility. They don't have duties.

Attendant García: A patient, if he's lucid, has to get up on time, wash himself, do the jobs assigned to him, and be obedient with the rest.

Attendant Hoyos: Behave himself and respect the nurses and the attendants, and especially the doctors.

Attendant Ibáñez: It seems to me that he doesn't have a duty, because you can't demand anything from him. Only the doctors have something to say. If they had a duty it would be to take their rest here in the pavilion.

Attendant Jiménez: Not to offend anyone or do any harm to anybody's health.

Attendant León: He should be obedient to a person, show respect. He should go to bed at bedtime, at 7.

Attendant Llona: He ought to know how to get along well with the attendants and the nurses. He shouldn't try to escape from the pavilion, so as to avoid bothering the nurses, as well as his relatives.

Attendant Meza: Of course, it's that he remain in the Hospital. The patient needs to cooperate with medications, with the nurses, doctors, and attendants. It's that they have a strange will, because they expect willingness from their relatives and the doctor's permission.

Attendant Nores: It would be to obey in what they're told, to take their pills when the nurse gives them out, and to eat their food.

Attendant Ortiz: Not to go outside the pavilion, just to be here when it's time for their medications.

Attendant Paredes: She should behave herself and enjoy her work. When she's better, she can help or to to *laborterapia*. They also have their club.

Interpretation

Interpretation of the data may be initiated with the observation that a transferred Hospital structure modeled on the Peruvian family is, indeed, to be found in the content of the interview responses, with the doctor playing the role of "father," the female nurse (along with the male nurse) acting as "mother," and the attendant assuming the position of "older sibling," all of them relegating the patient to the role of "younger sibling," possibly the "family's baby."[7] And it seems clear that the "parents" in this "family" have enormous power, as they do in North American hospitals. Stanton and Schwartz (1970:323) say in this regard: "The psychiatrist and nurse function not only as physician and nurse, but also as the government of the patients--executive, legislative, and judicial. They disburse economic favors, educate, chaperone and discipline, advise and protect."

Unconscious transference of figures who were of early significance in our lives to many social relations which we make later is a normal human psychological process. Klein (1975:48) states: "In some form or other transference operates through life and influences all human relations." It, therefore, is hardly surprising to find it in a psychiatric institution which, in that respect, is no different from any other human institution. What is *not* clear is the extent to which the actors in this family drama are aware of the roles they are playing--although these roles occasionally appear in the interview materials, possibly in a "preconscious" mode when some subjects use them as metaphors (including a male nurse who gave the nurse's role a "fatherly" significance). Let us review the materials.

The doctors see their role as connected to treatment of patients, and they define it as dedication to the latter with a constructive purpose; they also see themselves as resources for handling urgent situations on their services. Their duty is to understand mental illness, devote themselves to the evaluation of their patients so that they may get well, so that they may be restored to their groups or to society, or at least so that their capacities to engage in work be returned to them. Their responsibility is to "cure" in order to rehabilitate the curable ones or to maintain human levels of existence for the chronic ones. But doctors conceptualize good care in wider terms than the simple facts of understanding, supporting, and curing. Their duty includes research. And their responsibility extends beyond their relations with the patients to include the welfare of their services. A doctor has to make sure that his patients receive good treatment from everyone else in the hospital world; and, thus, he must provide orientation for other personnel, to motivate them.

Nurses, in contrast, say that the doctor should be punctual, come daily, go on his rounds and converse with his patients, be a serious man who makes everyone respect him, and have the initiative to improve the service. He should behave like a professional, be responsible, ethical, a gentleman, and love his work. Above all, the nurses emphasize, the doctor should collaborate with the nurse, work with the nurse in common accord; there should be comradely relations between the two, a lot of understanding. There are some doctors who abuse nurses by thinking that they are superior to them; but they ought to be considerate, have confidence in nurses, communicate with them, because the nurse is the doctor's right hand. A doctor has to control his nurse, but at the same time the nurses tend to agree that, while the doctor directs patient treatment, he has to inform them about it. The doctor should be concerned about his patients, their treatment, in order to watch for their recuperation, but he also has to see to it that the whole world of the service coperates toward that end.

For the attendants, the doctor ought to have a good manner with them, be frank with them, like them. He ought to be easy to get along with, not arrogant, and he should not fail to notice when an attendant greets him. He should show his kindness, his confidence in an inferior, and he should respond positively to requests for favors. He should be generous to humanity, and so he should be good to personnel as well as patients. He is responsible for the health of the whole world. He has to see to the progress of the service, the patients, the personnel and what they are doing, and go on rounds to make sure the patients are clean. At the same time, he is a being who is set apart because he has to know what is not known by the attendant. He has to direct the service with calm and peacefulness; but there also is a need to satisfy him: attendants have to be alert when he needs information in order to satisfy him with their answers.

The nurses see themselves as indispensable in the service (one says "like a father at home," but the role is more like that of a mother when others say "the doctor's first assistant" and "the doctor's right hand"--both conceptions possibly deriving from Nursing School indoctrination), as much for the doctors as for the patients and attendants. The nurse is responsible for the service, because the doctor only comes for a few minutes and does not stay for a long time. The nurse is the treatment base and without her or him things would not get done: without nursing there would be no medicine. The nurse has to see to discipline: she has to have things carried out, as well as to carry out things herself. The nurse collaborates with the doctor: she has to follow his orders, and she has to pass along to him her observations of the patients. She distributes work to the attendants, and she must watch them to make sure they obey. And she has, constantly, to see to the care of the patients, to help them, teach them how to live outside the Hospital when they are discharged (and doubtlessly within the Hospital as well), and she should make herself liked and respected by them so that they will obey her with affectionately.

The doctors also see the nurse as a helper: a nurse should cooperate with the doctor in the care and treatment of patients. She is like the doctor, but "within her professional sphere." The nurse has to obey the doctor's orders, discuss problems that come up, inform him about everything that happens among the patients, and, as some husbands may say about their wives, not create problems; or she should give care according to medical direction, according to the guides that the doctor gives her; and she should not get distracted by other things. A nurse has to be responsible for watching out for the service, from patients' comfort to preventing fights among them. She should slip around the service, doing her duties, softly and peacefully; and, one doctor says, she should "mend the holes," doubtlessly, in the pavilion fabric.

For attendants, nurses make sacrifices for the good of the service. Attendants have to be at their orders because nurses are the ones who assign work to them. Nurses can be rather strict, curt, and they scold attendants who come late, let patients out without telling them, or do not keep patients in good order. Sometimes they are condescending, despotic, and even blame attendents for their own faults. They ought to be less selfish and more friendly. Furthermore, like good mothers, they should be affectionate. They should be good persons who do favors for attendants, getting along well with and being kind to attendants and patients, respecting them and being respected. They should know an attendant and his or her circumstances. They should give explanations of how to deal with patients.

The attendants see themselves as workers, although they usually call themselves "employees." They define their role in terms of cleaning chores, having everything in place. They say that they are at the orders of doctors and nurses, and that they have to obey the orders of their superiors, carry them out. An attendant should collaborate with a nurse in looking after the patients, and so he is a help on the service. But the attendant has more contact with the patients than anyone else, and so it is his duty to protect them, care for them, watch them so as to stop fights and disagreements among them so they will not harm each other. In this sense, the function of attendants is control, but they also see themselves as helpers in psychiatric treatment.

The doctors define the role of attendants in terms of their primary functions: cleaning and vigilance (and, one adds, door-keeping), both non-medical labors, although some concede that attendants participate in therapy to some extent because they are present in the Hospital. Their participation in the service is seen to include the duties of caring for patients, treating them well, feeding them, getting them to participate in work, and collaborating or cooperating with doctors and nurses by informing them about what goes on in the service. The doctors see attendants as uncultured people but personnel who have direct dealings with the patients; therefore, they should understand patients better.

And the nurses offer a variety of observations on the attendants: they clean, bring food, take care of patients, in short, they do domestic service. Some are good, responsible, understanding, while others are careless or obtuse. They always have to be watched, because there are bad attendants who hit patients or insult them, or ones who are lazy, irresponsible, or slack in their work. They ought to know how to carry out their obligations, how to deal with, obey, and understand the nurse, respect their superiors, keep the service in order, be scrupulous with the patients, understand patients, be cooperative and efficient. Like the older children that a mother charges with the care of younger siblings, they need preparation for leading patients, and so it would be desirable to educate them; then the good ones would be capable of accepting the goals set by the nurses.

The patients are seen as the passive part of the Hospital's population. Some doctors view them as having no duties: duties are not to be demanded of patients because they have no sense of responsibility, because it depends on their critical capacity, or because they do not believe they are patients; or symptoms can consist of non-cooperation; or because of their need for care; or they receive more than they can give. Nevertheless, most of the doctors emphasize duties like accepting or receiving treatment, therapy, or the doctor's efforts, cooperating or collaborating with the doctor, submitting to treatment, or obeying orders or prescriptions. Some see the patient's duty as obeying the rules or following discipline, or collaborating in the work or the progress of the Hospital, while others say that a patient should get along well with paramedical personnel, try to understand his condition. communicate what he feels, or help other patients.

The nurses also define the patient's role in terms of carrying out, respecting, or accepting medical orders, although they add nurses' orders to those of doctors. They emphasize cooperation, obedience, and collaboration in treatment--allowing oneself to be treated. Some nurses place emphasis on respect: respecting personnel or the white coat, being respectful; while others emphasize the rules: submitting to or observing Hospital regulations, watching out for discipline, or doing what the Hospital has arranged for them, like eating, going to bed, being reachable, taking medicine, or being at the nurse's orders. Two nurses say that the patient has to know or to adapt, or adapt to circumstances; and one says that a patient in serious condition has no obligations.

The attendants place emphasis, as may be imagined, on the patient's duty to obey attendants, be obedient, follow attendants' orders, help in the work of the service, comply with getting up, going to bed, washing, eating, and taking pills at the right times, being grateful to attendants, respecting and getting along well with attendants, as well as with the nurses and doctors. Some say that patients should not offend anyone or do any harm, or that they should not hit other patients or try to escape. Three say that patients have no duties. In all of this the attendants appear to take the role of older siblings, charged by the parents with the care of their younger siblings.

The incompetent babies, i.e., the patients, from these points of view have no voice in these matters. Again, and here in the context of a different set of structures from those discussed in Chapter 2, patients appear to be cut off from any active role in their own therapy.

Conclusion

All of this is not to deny that apart from transference processes there exists a medical-psychiatric ideology in which, according to Erikson (1970:172),

> psychiatry has tended to visualize the human mind by the use of intricate structural analogies--beginning, perhaps, with Freud's use of topographical terms and continuing throughout a literature in which the ego is likened to a building or machine and disorder is likened to a failure of supports, a weakening or collapse of foundations, and so on. . . . Thus, it should be a matter of small surprise if the analogy is taken too seriously and patients enter the therapeutic setting with the passive attitude that they have come to be "fixed," or with the

> comfortable notion that mental illness is something which has "happened" to them, something in which they are only indirectly implicated, like an "enemy" invasion of germs.

Thus the passive role of patients is overdetermined, as are also the roles of the Hospital personnel, since they are all associated with Hospital ideology, not to mention associations with culture, social class and political economy.

Nevertheless, it may be maintained that structural transference is not without significance in what takes place in the Hospital. However, we still must ask not only if it is possible, in reality, to reproduce family structure in a mental hospital, but also if it is desirable. Rapoport (1960:72) makes the observation that

> it is clear that hospitals as at present constituted *cannot* reproduce identical patterns of relationships--e.g., family life. Furthermore, study reinforces the view that "too realistic" a confrontation of some patients with the characteristic problems and processes of ordinary life only exacerbates the difficulties initially stimulated outside the hospital. Patients, as casualties of the social processes in the world outside the hospital, may need *different* conditions in which to recover or to nurture their capacity to live with psychological or sociological comfort in ordinary society.

At the same time, as a prototype of all social relations, it may be contraindicated to conceive of the family model as antitherapeutic in itself. A. Freud and Burlingham (1943:156-161) discovered the advantages of "artificial families" in their work in a nursery with small children who were evacuated from London during World War II. Many of these children regressed under the stress of separation from familiar persons and surroundings. They resolved many such problems by subdividing the large group of children into small clusters around "substitute mothers," each one of whom had charge of her "family." They conclude:

> The occurrences in this group are . . . a clear demonstration of the known fact that children transfer their early relationship to their families onto all the people who later play an important part in their lives. This transference of feeling is responsible, on the one hand for the stormy and conflicting nature of the attachment of the child to the nursery worker, for the mixture of love and hate, possessiveness and

> jealousy. It explains, on the other hand, why the consequences of such attachments are so far reaching where education and development is concerned. With the full return to the type of attachment which had been interrupted by the separation from the family, the child resumes his steady progress towards the formation of a normal personality.

I do not assert that a nursery is the same as a psychiatric hospital. Still we can conclude, minimally, that it is not necessarily antitherapeutic as a model with which a hospital might construct a therapeutic program *to begin with*, although, perhaps, it may not be the goal, taking into account that in therapeutic activity the object is to emerge from transference, there being developed in the process the human capacity to participate in more differentiated and complex social relations, which for patients might mean getting well and for personnel might mean deliverance from "closet insanity." The transcultural study of the family informs us that a wide variety of family forms exists: while the family is universal, its content varies. Thus, there are tremendous possibilities for using the family model therapeutically. For example, we could ask, if there must exist custodial functions, then what kinds or qualities of custody might we choose from? What is intriguing, ultimately, is that these possibilities can take form in a situation where people who are aware that they are acting out family roles may choose to exercise control over them, in place of being controlled by them.

Notes

1. Role expectations among patients for themselves and others are treated in Chapter 4 and do not need to be repeated here. The doctors' points of view are explored in Chapter 1; the attendants' in Chapter 6; and the nurses' in Chapter 7.
2. Nurses Bustos, Cruz, Chivas, Esquivel, Hurtado, Losada, and Llosa are men; Nurses Arruga, Delgado, Frías, Godoy, Iglesias, and Justo are women.
3. All identities are fictitious. Names are assigned alphabetically according to the date of the interview, from September 29 to December 5, 1959.
4. Attendants Alfaro, Costa, Chacón, Durán, Estrada, Fuentes, García, Hoyos, Ibáñez, Jiménez, León, Llona, and Meza are men; Attendants Bravo, Nores, Ortiz, and Paredes are women.
5. A shop on the Hospital grounds in which charity patients produce articles

for sale, for the Charity Society's profit. I prefer to call it "labor therapy" rather than "occupational therapy" because any therapeutic benefit that might be derived by the patients who work there is accidental.

6. This series of responses about the patient's duty has been presented in summary form in Chapter 2. For the patient's point of view, see Chapter 4.

7. The lucid patients I interviewed, of course, did not see themselves as babies, although they appear to place personnel in the appropriate family roles. See Chapter 4.

Chapter 6

Deferred Hopes: The Psychiatric Attendants

This chapter reports on the interviews with attendants in the Hospital Victor Larco Herrera. The aim is to present a picture of the attendants in terms of what they said about their lives and their work in the Hospital, explore the possibilities of their more effective integration into their therapeutic labors, and to suggest some resistances that might appear between the rational search for this goal and its realization.

As an introduction to the materials, and before performing the tasks which have just been outlined, it will be useful to engage in a general examination of the position of attendant (or aide) within the structure of a psychiatric hospital. Belknap (1956:37-51) distinguishes three divisions or horizontal levels of this structure: a high level of professional persons, a middle level of administrators, and a low level of aides, nurses' aides, or workers, each one separated from the others by profound differences in rural vs. urban backgrounds, education, previous occupations, and age, differences which, following Derrida (1978), not only distinguish them by their *difference* but as well by their *deferral*, with which the higher status person suspends, postpones, puts off, condescends to, and subdues the lower status person.

Bockoven (1972:106) suggests that the attendant "occupies the most difficult and frustrating position" in the traditional asylum:

> He [or she] seves as guard and taskmaster whose duty it is to preserve order by restricting patients' spontaneous movements to a minimum and by closely supervising any duty he directs the patient to perform. He is the most important person in the patient's life, but his position in the hospital hierarchy is of the lowest order. He is subjected to a rigid discipline which requires him to maintain an impersonal relationship with patients and holds him responsible for any mishap which occurs. He must constantly be on the lookout lest some patient acquire a bit of glass, a length of rope, a sliver of wood, or a supply of matches; for every patient is suspect of harboring violent tendencies or desires to escape. He must even restrict conversation between patients lest altercations result. He is fulfilling his duties well if he is observed to be presiding over a scene of somber silence when the supervisor, nurse, or physician "trips" through his ward. All told, his task is a thankless one, for like the patient he remains in good standing only so long as there are no mishaps. There is no way he can progress or better himself. At best, his prospect is the monotony of uneventful life on a "well-managed" ward. . . . And in the public mind his capacity to endure close association with the fancied depravity of the mentally ill places him in a category as uniquely stigmatized as mental illness itself.

Belknap (1956:37-51) accurately distinguishes three *vertical* divisions of the structure: first, a division of psychiatric medicine; second, one of maintenance, which includes an administrator and administrative personnel; and third, a custodial one which includes attendants and their supervisors. The functioning of this third system, Belknap indicates, that of custodial supervision, is charged with the obligations "to receive and care for mental patients on a 24-hour basis in the wards, to establish routines for their deportment, health, dress, eating, and sleeping, to maintain maximum security for the patient and those around him." Without this "the hospital [would] collapse as an organized agency."

To illustrate the importance of the attendant in the hospital, Luchins (1959:78) asks his students of clinical psychology, rhetorically, "If all the doctors were to leave, what would happen to the hospital? Would it be able to function? Which functions would stop, which would be impaired, which would go on as before? . . . . What do you think would have the greatest influence on the hospital's functioning--if all the doctors left, if all the nurses left, or if all the aides left, and why do you think so?"

Parsons (1957:119) comments with regard to personnel categories of mental hospitals:

> There is . . . one category of great importance--because of contact with patients--namely the *attendant*. In terms of both qualifications and authority, his role is defined residually. He has responsibility in the direct care and management of patients, and yet he has no professional qualifications and no special competence other than that derived from direct experience. His role is clearly of great importance and because of the cost of professional personnel, a good deal of responsibility tends to be left in his hands. Until recently the role has often been defined mainly by practical exigencies rather than by any clear conception of positive function.

Attendants are effectively "paraprofessionals," those who work by the side of the professional person. Freidson (1970b:48-49) says:

> The term "paramedical" refers to occupations organized around the work of healing which are ultimately controlled by physicians. Physician control is manifested in a number of ways. First, much of the technical knowledge learned by paramedical workers during their training and used in their work tends to be discovered or enlarged upon or at the very least approved of by physicians. Second, the tasks performed by paramedical workers tend to assist rather than replace the focal tasks of diagnosis and treatment. Third, paramedical workers tend to be subordinate in that their work tends to be performed at the request or "order" of, and is often supervised by, physicians. Finally, the prestige assigned to paramedical occupations by the general public tends to be less than that to physicians. . . . These characteristics are such that the paramedical occupations may be distinguished from established professions by their relative lack of autonomy, responsibility, authority, and prestige.

Salisbury (1962:50-51) characterizes relations between doctors and attendants in the hospital he studied:

> The attendants are present on the ward, when a doctor comes visiting, but the doctor's main interest is in patients. Some attendants are efficient and some are not, and it is in terms of their efficiency in

> performing duties that doctors evaluate them. Attendants who quickly and accurately give the doctor the information he needs when asking questions are noticed, while those who do not, or who remain in the background, are ignored. If some accident happens, or if a patient escapes, the attendant on duty is called in by the doctor, who wants to find out what happened, and an inefficient attendant will be noted as such. . . . Since the reliable and efficient attendants are called in more often to give information, the doctor gets to know them better than the majority. Most of the other attendants the doctor does not even know by name, although, like any nominal superior dealing with a nominal inferior, he uses many devices to convince them that their feelings are considered.

Of the 448 persons classified as "workers" who were employed in the Hospital Victor Larco Herrera in 1959, almost half were occupied in the park, "labor therapy," and other tasks outside the pavilions. Only 258 worked in the pavilions in intimate contact with patients. These workers were diplomatically referred to as "*empleados*," "employees," by other personnel categories.[1] Pavilion 20 had 14 attendants, of whom I interviewed 13. 4 additional attendants were interviewed in other pavilions, making a total of 17, 13 men and 4 women.

The Peruvian attendant worked in an institution managed by the Public Charity Society of Lima, a bureaucratic organization that engaged in many other charitable and public service activities. As has been pointed out, what was noteworthy in this situation was that the doctors, who are necessary in a psychiatric hospital, were separate in the lines of power from the administration and did not have great influence in the management of the Hospital (or, at least, they did not have the influence they desired). Thus, even though the attendant was, as Freidson (1970a:144-145) observes, in a subordinate position to others' authority, subordinated as much to bureaucracy as to the alleged superior knowledge and judgment of professional persons, it would appear that he or she was less in Henry's (1954:141) situation of "multiple subordination," where the paraprofessional has more than one superior from whom to take orders. In the Lima Hospital, the line of authority was very clear from the point of view of the attendant: he or she received orders from the head of the service, the nurse, or from the Nursing Supervisors, who were authorities for the nurses, or even the Hospital administrator. Not one of 13 attendants I asked mentioned that he or she received orders from the doctors, although they all clearly recognized that they owed them great respect and even veneration.

We may begin the task of reviewing the attendants' responses to the questions in a list of 65 items,[2] by giving a brief description of each one of the subjects,[3] a summary of the first few questions which sought data on their personal characteristics:

Attendant José Alfaro: He is 27 years old. He was born in a small town in the Northern Highlands. He attended primary school up to the third year. His relatives are farmers. His father is a livestock breeder. He came to Lima nine years ago. He worked for six months in construction, and then three months in the X_____ Clinic which is for poor children; and then he spent two years as a waiter in a bar. Then he came to work here.

He came to work in the Hospital, he says, "because at the time I wasn't making very much and because it was steady work here. I got the job because they told me that they were hiring at this Hospital. I went to the police and they gave me my good conduct certificate. I said to myself that I was going to see if I could get one of those vacancies, and luckily they hired me. A cousin of mine who was working across the street, in the orphanage, told me that there were always openings. He told me to get my papers together and come and look at it."

He earns 60 pounds [*libras*, in Spanish, each equivalent to ten soles] a month. Sometimes, yes, his income is enough, and sometimes it isn't. He also has another job. He works as a cashier in a commercial house and earns a percentage. "Sometimes it doesn't pay, and other times I come out with 70 or 80 pounds. I have to pay rent for the house and support my family. I'm not married but I have a wife and two babies. My brother also lives with us. We're about six persons in the house. My brother is studying.

"I don't know if I'm going to stay here. It depends. I plan to stay for this year. If it gets better I'll stay for a few years. Otherwise, I expect to leave. My wife comes from a city on the North Coast. They have houses and fields there. I'm thinking of going there to be a farmer."

Attendant Carmen Bravo: She is 23 years old. She was born in a small town of the Northern Highlands. She has been in Lima for a year and nine months. Before, she was a teacher in a primary school on a rural estate in a coastal Department [a political subdivision of Peru]. She worked there for six years. Before that, she was in high school in the capital city of that Department. Currently, she is studying in a Lima high school. She just started.

Here in Lima she spent eight months in her sister's house. Her sister is a close friend of one of the doctors. The sister spoke with him so that Carmen could come to work in the Hospital.

She has been working here for eight months. She came here, she says, "because I liked nursing a lot and because there was that connection with Dr. Fernández. I began to work with him in Hospital Y_____. After two weeks, he moved here. I stayed there until he called me to come here."

She is making 74 pounds. She has no other job because she is going to school. She is single. Her income is enough because she lives with her brother and mother. She says, "If I get to finish my studies, I don't know what career would be the most comfortable for me. I'm thinking of staying here until I finish school. To get into nursing, a person has to be under 25, but I don't know if I'll get finished with school in time. A person can start in the fifth year of high school, but I just began. Then there are six years of nursing to do."

Attendant Enrique Costa: He is 22 years old. He was born in a small town in the Central Highlands. His primary education was to the fifth year. He came to Lima a year and three months ago. Before that, he lived for two years in a small city on the Central Coast. Then he went back to the Central Highlands, to a large city where he worked as an assistant in a carpentry shop. Then he changed to a mining compamy where he worked in the construction of a tunnel. His family is in the livestock business back home. His father is dead. He had been a teacher in primary school for twenty-eight years.

He says, "I got the job here through a relative who worked here. I applied, but I had to wait three months. I was looking for work all over Lima. I came to work here because there weren't any other economic opportunities. He earns 750 soles a month. "It's enough. I'm single, no woman. I have to help my younger brothers and my mother. They're in the Highlands. I live here in my aunt's house."

He has no other job. He says, "I think I'll stay here for a while until I can find some regular job. Next year I want to go to high school. I expect to stay in the Hospital until I'm done with school. I'd like to be a professional, working in an ordinary profession like mechanics."

Attendant Manuel Chacón: He is 23 years old. He was born in a small town in the Northern Highlands. He was in primary school to the fourth year. He has been a laborer, student, and "farmer helping my father." He came to Lima directly from his town seven years ago. He says, "I came to work here on October 15, 1954, and I worked till

July 31, 1955. Then I went on active service in the Air Force for two years. Next I worked for another year apart from here. I worked in the fields, doing construction, everything. Then I came to work here for the second time on August 1, 1958."

He is making 62 pounds a month with a bonus of S/.144.70. He says, "The government is giving us the bonus. A basic wage hasn't been established yet. Yes, I work outside here, but it's not stable and I do it when I can. I do painting. Sometimes I work for two or three days a week, and other times I don't. Sometimes I work till 11 or 12 at night. That's when there's a lot of work. I work maybe ten to fifteen days a month. I earn 20 or 30 soles a day. That's barely working for a kilo of meat. Rice has gone up to 3.30. Poor people don't eat meat."

He came to work in the Hospital "because there was the convenience that they feed us here. It's also easy work. It's steady work. I like it for the convenience." After he got his certificates, he waited two months to go to work. He adds, "Before, I had an uncle who worked here. He told me it would be good to work here, because it was hard outside, and here there was food which a person didn't get on the streets." He is not satisfied: "Prices have gone up and what you earn is so little. I'm trying to find other work. I'd like to be a policeman. Maybe some time I'll be able to study for it. If I get accepted into the Police regiment, in a month, I'll get out of here. I'd like to be a policeman, and to study, too. I hope I can rise in the world that way. Otherwise, I'd like to be a practical nurse. In the Police Hospital they call practical nurses "sanitarians" and nurses "graduates." I'd like to be a policeman so I could begin studying, because a person gets advanced in the entrance examinations for the officers' school."

Attendant Francisco Durán: He is 21 years old. He was born in a small town in the Northeast Highlands. He has completed four years of primary school. Soon he will have been in Lima for a year. He came directly from home. There, he says, "I worked doing chores in my parents' house, in farming, and doing a little carpentry. I came to stay in Lima a while, to get to know it and to see if anything would turn up for me, but if not, to go back home."

He has worked here between four and five months. He says, "One of my brothers was working here and he told me about it. I came to see Señorita Mendoza. I was living in Lima with him. I'd been here applying to the Police School. They threw me out in the last examination." He is earning 60 pounds and, with the bonus, it comes to 70. It's enough because he is single. He does not work outside the hospital but takes care of his brother's house.

He plans to continue working here, he says, "as long as God helps me. I'm not sure. I'm thinking about going to high school so I can look for an opening. Maybe I'll start next April."

Attendant Carlos Estrada: He is 30 years old. He was born in a small town in the Northern Highlands. He went to primary school through the third year. He has been in Lima for eight years. He came here after he finished his military service in the Air Force near a city on the North Coast. He worked in a restaurant as a cook's helper. Later he was a chef. "Then I applied for work in the orphanage across the street which also belongs to the Charity Society. I worked there for around a year and then I applied here. I came to work here because there I was working all day, and here it's just half a day. Then you can look for a little job outside." A friend who worked here advised him to make the change.

When he came, he earned 18 pounds, the same as in the orphanage. Now he get 740.75, with the bonus. He comments, "The wage isn't enough because I have a family." Yes, he works outside, "in gardening. I'm a gardener in private houses here in Magdalena [the part of Lima in which the Hospital is located] from 3 to 5 p.m., sometimes till 6. Some days you make some money and others you don't. It depends if you find work. I make between 10 and 15 pounds a month, 20 to 30 soles for an afternoon." He is married, and there were five children. One died and now there are four, at the ages of 5, 4, 3, and the baby who is 3 months old.

He plans to remain in this job, but "it depends on whether they increase the wage a little bit. Otherwise, I'd like to go back home, maybe after a couple of years. I'd work at whatever job paid the most. I'd work double, hard, to make some money."

Attendant Luis Fuentes: He is 23 years old. He was born in a small town in the Central Highlands from where he came to Lima 4 years ago. He has five years of primary schooling. After he was settled in Lima, he says, "I worked in a private home doing domestic service. I worked that way for a year. Then I came to work here in the Hospital. I came because I was making very little out there, and here you make a little more. I got the job through a friend. He recommended me. He was working here. He still does. He's a nurse. He told me how much you got here and advised me to come. My relatives live far away. They say I should keep on working but not to stay too long."

He makes 60 pounds a month. The income is more or less enough "to pay rent and expenses." He lives alone. He does not have a woman or children, and he is not engaged. He has another job outside, he says," in a truck. I'm a truck driver. It's a private truck. A man who comes from my town is the owner. I work from 5 in the morning to 10, all week long, 7 days, and I make 30 pounds. [I comment about his earnings of less than 10 soles an hour, something less than 40 U.S. cents at the time.] It's dangerous work and you have to be careful. We're very backward here in Peru."

He does not expect to continue his work in the Hospital. He says, "It depends. I'm planning to study this year in a private high school. I want to study mechanics. The course is for two years. So I'm going to work here at least two years till the course is over. I'll have to do everything possible to pay for school expenses."

Attendant Alberto García: He is 20 years old. He was born in a small town in the Central Highlands. He has a secondary school education to the third year, which he is in "right now." His examinations begin at the end of this month [November]. He is going to continue in the fourth year, next year. He says, "I came here to study through the fourth year." First he went to another city on the Central Coast, and then he came here. His grandfather is there. He explains, "I had an uncle who worked here, before. I came to Lima to go to high school, but because I was 16 years old I couldn't be admitted in the day session because the age limit was 15. I had to go to night school. I didn't work during the first year. I stayed home during the day and spent the time studying. Because I had time and because my uncle was there, he advised me to come here. It's convenient because I work in the morning, study in the afternoon, and go to school at night, from 8 to 11. That's from Monday to Friday. On Sunday mornings there's an obligatory course in military instruction. I told my uncle that I wanted to work here because I had the whole day free. I also wanted to work here because I live in Magdalena, very close, and I don't have to worry about transportation. My father sends money to the six of us who are here. He's going to come to take two of us back there for the vacation. They're also going to high school. I'm going to stay and work, but when I have my vacation I'm going back home too. My relatives have been telling me to look for a better job. This atmosphere doesn't help you to learn."

He has been working in the Hospital for a year and seven months. He makes 600 soles a month. He is single, not engaged. He adds, "Life is dear in Lima. A friend of mine in the Central Post Office told me I ought to come to work there as an employee, because we get workers' wages here. But the hours weren't convenient: from 8:30 to 12 and 3:30 to 8, and my school begins at 8. It's worth the trouble to finish high school and then look for another job. I'd like to continue in higher education. I like science in general. We have lands in my town and I'd like to be an engineer-agronomist."

Attendant Nestor Hoyos: He is 24 years old. He was born in a small town in the Northeast Highlands. He has a primary education up to the third year. Before he came to Lima, six years ago, he was in school and then working in the fields at home. He says, "When I came to Lima I worked for two years in a laundry. Then I worked in a hardware store for a year. I was a clerk. Then I got sick. I left that job and I stayed out for six months. Next I looked for work in a chemical company. I worked in the warehouse opening cans and unloading trucks that brought things that came from foreign parts. I worked like that for three months and then I came here. I came because they were paying a little more, so I could lead a little better life, and because transportation was easier. I don't have to pay carfare because I live close by."

He has been working in the Hospital for a year and five months. He got the job, he says, "through the intervention of one of the people from my home town who works here. I asked him as a favor to help me to get this job. He spoke with the head of personnel. Then they made an appointment for me to come to the office. I didn't have to wait because there were openings."

He earns 742 soles a month. He has no outside job. He explains, "In my free time I read my books and notes from my studies so I won't forget. I'm planning to go to school next year to finish primary school and, if God wants it, to go on with high school." He is not married but he has a companion and one baby of 10 months. Yes, the income is enough, "because I live with a friend in a room. We only pay a little for the room, 80 soles. My friend helps with the expenses. We pay half-and-half. I don't know, frankly, if I'm going to continue working in the Hospital. I'm ready to look for a better job and get out. I'm looking around right now. More or less I've found some possibilities. A person wants a little better wage to live more comfortably. I'd like to be a mechanic. I'm hoping to enter a technical school."

Attendant Pablo Ibáñez: He is 22 years old. He was born in a small town in the Central Highlands. He went as far as the first half year of high school. He says, "I came to Lima when I was a boy. I've been here for seven years. I came here to work. I was a chicken dealer in the Central Market between 1952 and 1954. In 1954 I had a quarrel with a man that I worked with, and so I went into a business with a relative. He was a bird dealer too. I worked like that for six months. Then I had some brothers who were working in an insurance company. I worked there a year as a barber. I didn't like the work and they were paying very little. I left and went to work in construction. In 1955, after six months, I came here to work. I got my papers ready but they didn't put me to work till March of 1956. I have a cousin who was working here. He recommended me."

He earns 60 pounds a month with a bonus of 14 1/2 pounds. "I came here because it made it a little easier to work outside too. I'm a wholesaler. I work as a specialist in notions like silk ribbons, all kinds of colored remnants, decorations for women's blouses. I sell them in the market. It's the only outside work I have. I do two shifts here and when I have a free day I go to Paramonga or Huacho [coastal cities north of Lima], to the markets there. That's on Saturdays, but on Sundays I have to work here. This morning I went to the market in Callao [Lima's port]. Tomorrow afternoon I'm going to work somewhere else. I don't know where I'm going to go, maybe to a wholesale house. I keep my accounts in a book. I have to collect from my clients each month. I earn around 90 pounds, aside from capital.

"The income isn't enough. I'm married, with a baby of 5 months. Our house costs 25 pounds. Then there's light and taxes for the police and the street. I don't buy meat here but in Huaral. We buy enough for two weeks. My wife's in business too. She sells the same things that I do, but retail. I'm thinking about leaving Lima in 1962 to to to C_____ [a highland city] to open a radio shop. I left high school and entered a technical school where I studied for two years. My cousin has a shop. Sometimes I go there to help him. But I want to work on my own account. I need to get some capital to get out of here, and I'll be ready in 1962. I picked C_____ because I like it. I've gone there on business. I went one week during my vacation. I have a brother-in-law who used to work there. My wife is from a city on the South Coast."

Attendant Tomás Jiménez: He is 21 years old. He was born in a small town in the Northern Highlands. He was in a commercial secondary school to the third year. He came to Lima 10 years ago straight from his home town. He came because he was brought by his family. He explains, "First I worked in an accounting firm. I left there for military service. When I got out of that, five months ago, I came to work here. My father works in the orphanage across the street. He knew Señor Mendoza and they arranged for me to come and work here. Currently I'm studying in a technical school. This year I'll finish radio, and next year I'll be in television. I'm working here to pay the expenses of my studies. I asked Señor Mendoza if I could work in the office, and he told me that I could work here until there was a vacancy."

He is earning 740 soles a month. He has no wife and is not engaged. His income is enough to pay for his studies. He says, "I live with my parents and brothers and sisters close by here. I plan on staying on here till March 1960, because then I'll be finished with radio. I'm planning on setting up a shop. I'll keep on with advanced studies in television and electronics. I want to have my shop and buy a house."

Attendant Jorge León: He is 27 years old. He was born in a small town in the Northeast Highlands and came to Lima four years ago. He has all six years of primary school. He says, "First I worked in a stable. It was like a cattle ranch. I worked there nine months. It was all right. There was food and a bed inside. Then I left that and went to work in a metal carpentry shop. It was when they closed the stable and nine of us had to leave. In the new job we made doors and windows. I worked there for a year and a half. Then I came here. I came because the work I was doing wasn't steady. It was just for periods of time. This work was steadier. I came here with the help of a gentleman who knew me, just a friend. He was working in the Hospital."

He is earning 61 pounds a month with a bonus of 13. He does not have an outside job, but he is thinking about it. He says, "In my free time I wash clothes and visit my relatives. I'm single but engaged. We still haven't fixed a date. We have to have a budget. We have a child 2 years old. Sometimes my income is enough and sometimes we need more. We live near the Hospital."

He does not plan to return to his home town. He states, "I want to stay at least a couple of years so as to get to know it, unless some misfortune happens to us if we don't have what we need. Then we could go back home. I have lands there. My relatives are farmers. After a couple of years, I'd like to move to the Hospital Dos de Mayo, because you learn more there than you do here. I'd like to be a practical nurse, and here that possibility doesn't exist. I have three cousins who are working there. One cousin might go to the Police Hospital. I have another cousin who works there. I went there seven times to apply, but I couldn't get in because there was no vacancy. There are many opportunities to practice this profession back home.

There are hospitals, and a person can work in private homes."

Attendant Augusto Llona: He is 24 years old. He was born in a small town in the North-Central Highlands. He has six years of primary schooling. He has been in Lima three times. He explains, "I came here in 1951 and went back in 1954. I came the first time because of my father's illness. I spent the whole time in the Hospital Dos de Mayo, staying with my father. I had a place to stay, but the Mother Superior gave me a bed there in the hospital. I couldn't work because my father couldn't be alone. His face was covered with bandages. I had to feed him. We went back home and he died in 1955, after a year. The doctors had done everything possible to cure a swelling he had on his face.

"Then I came back here in 1957. First I went to another city on the Central Coast where I worked as a waiter in a bar. Then I came here in 1958. After I arrived in Lima I was working in a gasoline station. I did that for six months while I was applying to come to work here in the Hospital. I wanted to work here because they weren't paying us enough there, and besides I have a family and the wages weren't enough. Here you earn a little more than there. I got the job through my brother-in-law who works here in the Hospital. He was looking out for me, and when the day came that there was a vacancy, he told me. I've been working here for 6 months.

"Here I get 600 soles with a bonus of 145. I don't have an outside job. I'm married with two children, a boy and a girl. The little boy is 2 years and 8 months, and the baby is 6 months old. We live close by with my two brothers-in-law, and the wife of one of them who is married. We share expenses. I go back home in the afternoon to take care of the baby. My wife works. She's an assistant to a dress-maker. She earns 10 soles a day, from 2 in the afternoon to 7. She just started, and when you are a beginner that's the wage. I didn't have another job before. It's very hard to find work. Our income is more or less enough because there are several of us together.

"I don't have a time set for staying in this job. It could be for a few years. I'd like to work for a while. Later I'd like to learn the tailoring trade. I have some ideas about that. I know how to make trousers. I still don't know how to make jackets. I learned back home. One of my uncles taught me. I want to learn the trade here. I can get into a school for men's clothing. Then I plan to return home where I have land."

Attendant Germán Meza: He is 33 years old. He was born in a small town in the Northern Highlands. He has three years of primary education. He has been in Lima five years. Before he came, he worked in the fields. He says, "I came here to work, because I had a brother who was working here and still does. In those days there were very few attendants, so there were vacancies. My brother wrote me about it, so I came to visit, to look at it and see if I could find a way of getting used to it. I took the job because it was a little more convenient. When you work a half day there's time to do personal things. I work outside at tailoring. I'm only like a worker. It's private work from 9 in the morning to 12 on most days. I'll finish my contract as an apprentice and then I can think about working on my own account. I had to pay for the school and I haven't earned anything yet."

He is making 60 pounds a month with a bonus of 143. His income is not enough. He explains, "It's necessary to sacrifice a little. We are renting in a *quinta* [an enclosed block of apartments around a courtyard]. There's my mother and brothers, four of us. Only one of my brothers is married. We share expenses because we're together. The whole weight isn't just on one. I'm single but I have my companion and two children of 2 months and 3 years. I have two more back home. I'm planning to work here for about two or three more months. It's a kind of low work. I don't know what's going to happen. I want to work in tailoring. It's working on your own, for yourself."

Attendant Ana Nores: She is 25 years old. She was born in a small town in the Southern Highlands from where she came to Lima 9 years ago. She has five years of primary schooling. She applied for a job in the Hospital seven years ago, she says, "because I needed to work. It was a little hard to find in other places, and I needed help because I was studying dress-making. I met a woman in class who was working here. We talked about it, and so I came with my papers to apply. My friend is still working here."

She earns 700 soles a month with the bonus. She also works at home, "when people who know me give me orders for sewing. It's not a definite thing, but something that happens now and then. Some months I don't do anything. I work eight hours here and I'm not doing dress-making. If there's time, I can earn 30 soles in two or three days. I'm single. I'm engaged but not married. I have three children of 5, 2, and 5 months. The head of the house is an assistant investigator, a policeman, like a detective. He is making 1,600. We're living with his mother, my mother-in-law. Sometimes it seems to us that our income is enough, but other times the children get sick, and so sometimes we have serious difficulties. The head of the house can rise a little, but he can't be a chief because a chief has to have higher education. It's a military matter. It depends on luck.

"My father wants me to learn something so I can work elsewhere. He is hoping that some day I'll find better work. He wants me to go back home to work as a practical nurse. Or I could move to the Hospital Obrero, or Militar, but those jobs are hard to get.

"It's difficult working away from home but the situation doesn't allow anything else. My mother-in-law takes care of the children. I couldn't say how long I'm going to keep on working here, because if I can find a situation where I can earn a little more I'll have to get out of here. I'm waiting for the baby to grow a little more before I apply for another job. I'd like to work at dress-making or practical nursing, or be a nurse's aide. There's a three-month course in the Hospital Empleado. At Obrero you learn according to your capacity. Here there's no nurse's aide. We do everything."

Attendant Luisa Ortiz: She is 30 years old. She was born in the capital city of a Department in the Northeast Highlands, from where she came to Lima fifteen years ago. Her schooling was to the second year of primary here in Lima. She worked for three years in the Z_____ Clinic. Before that, she worked in a doctor's house. She says, "They brought me up like I was their daughter. I worked there about five years. I went to work in the Clinic because the doctor returned to the highlands and I stayed in Lima to work. I came to the Clinic to make my application. There wasn't any other job. I asked the administrator if there were vacancies. I had a cousin who worked there and she told me what the service was like, how the patients were. Now she's back in the highlands. The lady who hired personnel in the Clinic also worked here. She asked me if I wanted to come here to work."

She earns 72 pounds a month including the bonus. She has never worked outside, because with "working two shifts here there hasn't been time." Currently, she says, "I'm studying dress-making as an apprentice. I study from 5 in the afternoon to 7. It's in a primary school. I have to pay for it. The supplies cost 150 for the whole course. It's a three-year course and I've just started the first year. I like to do dress-making and repairs because it's all different.

I'm single but engaged. We don't have children. My man works in a gasoline station. He earns 800 a month. Our income is enough. We live in a *quinta* with relatives and we share the expenses. Everything is expensive now. I plan to stay here three or four years more. If God permits me to learn to sew I'll work as a dress-maker. That way a person can work at home on her own account.

> Attendant Yolanda Paredes: She is 28 years old. She was born in a small town in the North-Central Highlands. Her primary schooling was complete. She came from home to Lima in 1950, she says, "because I wanted to work to help my mother. I came here to the Hospital because a friend of mine was working here, and through her I got this job. I will be here eight years on January 3."
>
> She makes 60 pounds a month, 70 with the bonus. She does not have another job. She complains, "The wages aren't enough. There are so many things to buy. I'm single, not engaged. I live with my sisters. There are six of us. They're married and have children. I'm the only one who's single. I'd like to save up something so I could get out of here, so I could look for another job, some trade, something like that. I'd do anything, maybe some kind of business. We'd be at peace. I'd like to open a fruit stand if an opportunity presented itself."

While these attendants hoped to better themselves economically, as is clear in the interview materials, it also appears that they were very glad to have steady work, with social security and union benefits, in a national context where unemployment and worker protection were a very serious problems, as is still the case today. Certainly, it was not possible for them to get their jobs in the Hospital without the intervention of relatives or friends who were already working there, who told them about vacancies and spoke with the administration in favor of the applicants. This was also a happy circumstance for the Hospital, it may be added, because thereby it could control a little more the quality of new attendants. Thus, the attendants had good reason to congratulate themselves for having good luck--even when they did not plan to remain on the job after they found something better which, for most of them, meant working on their own account as petty commodity producers. In relation to all this, Glaser (1963:55-57), speaking of the international variation in the discontent of health-related auxilliary personnel, in which North American attendants must occupy a very high, if not the highest, rank, suggests that "hospital employees in most countries are more satisfied than North American ones." This derives, according to this author, from a constellation of factors which include economic facts, because in many other countries "hospital work is a better job" because other good jobs are scarce, the differences in wages and other benefits between different jobs are small, and hospital employment has more prestige than most other workers' jobs. Also, doctors are not so busy and do not demand as much from their subordinates. Moreover, there are cultural motives, as for example in the competitive struggle of individuals for success. In Peru, workers with regular work have reason for satisfaction as they gaze at so many others, so much more unfortunate. Discontent, indeed, exists but it appears to be directed in the interviews at the economy in general more than at the Hospital.

Robinson (1964:209) observes that possibilities for attendants' advancement are few. Among Peruvian attendants such aspiration does not exist. An individual can only hope, as has been indicated, some day to work for himself/herself. Therefore, although there existed a turnover of the Hospital's personnel, it would appear that in comparison with hospitals in the developed world this did, and does, not occur with the same frequency. Grob (1983:19) notes the high rate of personnel turnover in North American psychiatric hospitals, the consequence of "long hours, arduous obligations in services filled with difficult patients, and relatively low wages." However, many of the Peruvian attendants indicated that their schedules were convenient or that their labors in the Hospital were easier than in many outside jobs. Grob (1991:120), in a more recent work, also notes the low quality of attendants as "perhaps the most serious problem that confronts mental hospitals." In contrast, in Peru attendants constituted a part of the labor elite, educated and with relatively good incomes, and with benefits most other workers lacked.

Let us now turn to the vision of the attendants themselves regarding their jobs, beginning with a question that was not as successful in eliciting "vision" as it was in obtaining an ethnographic description of the job from one of them. I asked my panel, 15. "How is the job of attendant here in general?" Most of the subjects responded with stereotypes phrases, but that one, Attendant Ibáñez, gave me a detailed description of the shifts. Only a selection of the responses which have illustrative value are presented here:

> Attendant José Alfaro: In a way we keep on doing the same job. It doesn't matter how many years you work, you don't advance. In Dos de Mayo there are practical nurses but we don't have that here.

> Attendant Enrique Costa: It's like domestic service. Yes, I'm satisfied.

> Attendant Francisco Durán: It's calm, pleasant.

Attendant Alberto García: I almost don't like it because it's a little disturbing for a person.

Attendant Nestor Hoyos: Fine. The wage is the only thing. All right, the food is also bad. Sometimes they send us the same kind of food that the patients get, with no meat. They fix very good food for the doctors.

Attendant Pablo Ibáñez: We come at 6:30 and report to the nurse. She gives us the stations where we are to work. Then we do cleaning in the stations she assigns us. We clean up and when everything is finished we rest a while. Then we tell the nurse that it's ready and she gives us another job. Sometimes it's going to the drug dispensary. Then they tell us to bathe the patients. Then it's time for lunch and we have to serve it to the patients. Then we clean up the pantry and soon it's time for the other shift. We rest till 1:30 and we report to the afternoon nurse. He tells us to leave our station clean. We do the cleaning and we get out at 2:30.

For the afternoon shift, we report at 12:30. The nurse tells us to clean the windows and wash the floors. Then we give the patients tea and we do cleaning again. We keep on till dinner. We serve the food again, do cleaning, and keep at it till 7. Everything is done and we get the patients ready to go to bed. We take off their clothes. Then we count the patients. The watchman comes and we give him the number. We do inspection with him and the nurse.

The watchman guards the patients all night to see that they stay in bed. He has a special noteook where he writes down what the patients do at night, the ones who walk around, those who don't sleep. The watchman makes sure they don't get into fights. If they get sick, he calls the nurse. He stays till 6:30 in the morning, until the morning nurse comes, when he hands over the service. The watchman has to deliver a clean pavilion to the morning personnel, so he has cleaning to do during the night. There's no vacancy now for working at night. I'd kind of like it. It's nice. I'd rather work at night, so I could do other things in the daytime.

Attendant Tomás Jiménez: It's like a worker. I'm going to keep on working the way I'm doing. It's good because it gives me the means to continue with my studies.

Attendant Luisa Ortiz: We do everything. We don't just have one job. We take care of the patients, as the nurses order. It's the way I'm working now.

> Attendant Yolanda Paredes: We take care of the patients, make their beds, bring food to them, wash them. We do the cleaning, too. That's the way we are. We're used to it. There isn't any other work. I don't like it.

While some attendants responded in a reserved manner to the questions, 22-24. "What are the attendant's duties?", "Which do you like most?", and "Which do you like least?", some gave responses which further brought to light an ethnography of the pavilions from the attendants' point of view. They revealed, as well, some of the attendants' reflections on their position in the Hospital's social structure. Here we are approaching a view of the Hospital's resistance to the use of attendants in a therapeutic role, a resistance not only stemming from unconscious processes going on in human minds but as well from social processes of which the actors are equally unaware. The attendants placed emphasis on their duties which had to do with cleaning and other physical tasks, and also on their roles as watchers and guards, to the complete exclusion of any therapeutic activity with patients. It can be said that they expected passively to receive and obey orders from their superiors:

> Attendant José Alfaro: When a person comes to work, he does it according to what the nurse orders him to do. When they say to clean this, he has to do it and have it clean and in good condition at the right time. He has to attend doctors' rounds when the nurse isn't there. He has to be at their orders. And then he has to go and get medications from the dispensary.
>
> The work I like is practice for spending my life a little more peacefully, in order to learn something. Here an attendant can't practice and learn anything. I'd like to work in mechanics or carpentry. You can learn how to do the cleaning in two or three days. In carpentry you don't learn much at the start, but when you do learn, the work turns out in good condition and you earn something and know something.
>
> I can't say that there's something I don't like, because all the services are the same.

> Attendant Enrique Costa: You do the cleaning in the pavilion, help in treatments, and obey the nurses' orders.
>
> I like everything. Everything's the same.

> Attendant Manuel Chacón: The duties are to take care of the

patients, feed them, help the nurse give them medicine, go to the pharmacy for medications. The whole service that's done in this pavilion is to be on watch here.

Since it's all work, all the tasks are the same for me. We don't have a specific job.

I don't like night work.

Attendant Francisco Durán: I have to carry out my duties as the boss, the nurse, orders. It's cleaning. It's also helping the patients, taking care of them with greater interest. And being here at the assigned hours.

For me all the duties are the same.

Attendant Carlos Estrada: When I arrive at 6:30, I give out clothes to the patients. After that I do the cleaning assigned to me. I make the beds for electroshock treatment. Then there are invoices for getting kerosene, DDT, rags, razor blades. It depends on orders from the nurses. We have to ask them to send us monthly soap, brooms, brushes, notebooks, fly swatters, toilet paper, liquid wax. We get all that from the dispensary on the 15th of the month. I also help with electroshock treatments, sometimes with insulin when there aren't enough personnel. Also in the pantry.

I like everything.

Attendant Luis Fuentes: You have to see to the service and the patients. You give them care, feed them, do services when the nurse tells you, make the beds, and see that they don't fight with each other.

In general it's all the same.

Attendant Alberto García: I work in the insulin therapy[4] room. Before that, we have to get the patients up at 6:30 so they can inject the insulin. Then we have to take them to bed so they can rest. They give the insulin in the nurses' station and we take them back to the room again. After that, we have to watch them in the precoma to see that they don't fall. We make a "cradle" [i.e., wrap a patient with sheets] when a patient is a little disturbed. Then comes the coma which lasts an hour. We have to watch so they don't have attacks of convulsions, because they can bite their tongues or do themselves some other harm. Then we begin to cut it with glucose. Syrup with milk is given to them with two pieces of bread, and then they get their clothes. Then it's time to take them to lunch. If a patient doesn't eat after he's cut, the coma can come back in the afternoon. At 12:30 we eat and at 1 we rest until 1:30. We report to the nurse and keep on working till 2:30. My job is cleaning the nurses' station.

I like work in the nurses' station because you get to clean everything, all the things we use in treatment.

I don't like the pantry and outpatient treatment. In the pantry we have to give out food and then clean up again. With outpatients, we have to take them to their beds. I prefer working in the insulin room because a person can learn a little more by watching the nurses and the doctors.

Attendant Nestor Hoyos: You have to come on time, obey punctually, do the cleaning correctly, and pay attention to the nurse when she calls and wants something.

I like to have my station clean, for example, to have the pantry clean. That's always my station. I don't like to be in the bathrooms for cleaning. I find them very dirty. There's vomit. It just happens sometimes, not every day, but you have to do it if that's your job.

Attendant Pablo Ibáñez: We're at the nurse's disposal.

We can't say that we don't like it. It's all the same. I like doing the cleaning.

There's no job I especially don't like.

Attendant Tomás Jiménez: We have to carry out our obligations as attendants in the Hospital, for example, to have everything in order in the station that belongs to a person. A station is a department for cleaning and watching the patients. Here the stations are the first room, the insulin room, the last room for physical therapy, the clothing room, this office [the room in which interviews were conducted], the nurses' station, the dining room, the doctors' offices, the patio, the second floor, and the basement. The outpatient room and the pantry don't have numbers, nor the corridors and the bathrooms. You have to lend a hand when there's outpatient treatment. We also have to help in the dining room and serve the patients. When a patient is disturbed, we have to try to make it so that he calms down and rests in bed. That's all.

I like to help with outpatient treatment when they give them injections, and in electroshock. It's more peaceful, calmer. This work is not very heavy. It's easier to work than in other stations.

I don't like it when they send us to take care of patients who are dangerous when they're disturbed.

Attendant Jorge León: You do your cleaning and see that everything is in good condition. If something's wrong, you tell the ones who can fix it. Even when you're cleaning they dirty it up, especially the corridors. Sometimes I'm on duty in the insulin room, or in electroshock, or I go to the pharmacy.

All the work looks the same to me. I go anywhere when they tell me to, and I do everything. It's all the same. I do everything with pleasure. I don't choose my station. Some attendants choose their stations, especially in the summer, but it's not important to me.

Attendant Augusto Llona: They change our work around. Sometimes I do cleaning in the corridors or the bathrooms. Other times I work in the dining room, or I watch the patients so they don't escape when I'm doing cleaning in the patio. I shave them too. I help in the insulin room and also in electroshock every Tuesday and Friday. I have to bathe the patients on Saturday afternoons, and also on Monday mornings. We give baths every Saturday, and just those on insulin on Mondays. After they bathe we give them a change of clothing. We put their clothes on, and their shoes. We tie the laces. We go to the pharmacy, the laboratory, the kitchen. We take them to the *kiosko* [a central coffee shop for patients who can leave their pavilions].

Everything seems easy to me. It's all the same. The bathrooms are a little unhygienic. I like taking them to the *kiosko* or going to the kitchen. I like taking care of the patients, serving them food.

Attendant Germán Meza: Each attendant has a station that he takes care of. If it's a room on the first floor, the first thing I have to do is to see that the patients are in good condition and are clean. In the second place, I do the cleaning that needs to be done and see that everything is in order. And I have to see that they don't fight with each other. Some of them are normal and others are in a state where they aren't aware. We have to make them a little calmer. In insulin therapy it's another kind of work, very different from work in the other rooms. That attendant has to take care of all the ones in daily treatment. There's one nurse and one attendant. Others help at certain times. Then the nurse is not alone with his eight or nine patients. In the past there used to be two rooms, but now there's just one upstairs. The students come for a few hours, and now we have women students. They just come during their practice months. A person is comfortable with everything, with all that has to be done. You don't choose. They order you, and you do what they tell you. Some stations are good and others are bad, but attendants change from one to the other. Most of my companions like to be in the patio to enjoy themselves and to be outside in the air. Clino-therapy is a little harder. They are immobile patients, in their beds. They can't eat and we have to feed them and move them. They aren't aware of anything any more.

Attendant Ana Nores: I do labor therapy. I watch that the patients work. I give them examples. I watch them constantly because being patients they can do anything that occurs to them. Sometimes they think of doing something they shouldn't be doing. In other stations I have to see to the patients, so that they eat, they have lunch, that the service is in order. You watch that they go to bed. I don't help in the insulin room or with electroshock because those are done in the morning.

I can't choose tasks because they rotate. I like doing labor therapy. I prefer tasks like that.

Attendant Luisa Ortiz: The duty is doing the cleaning, bringing the food to patients, carrying out orders from the nurses. That's our duty. I do the cleaning in this part, and I take care of the patients' relatives. I work in the clothing room. I don't work in the shop.

We have to like it. Some do insulin therapy, others clino-therapy in the rooms of disturbed patients. That's the way it is. We can't choose. The service is the same for everybody.

Attendant Yolanda Paredes: The duty is taking care of the service, seeing to whatever station it's our turn to care for, according to what the nurse orders us to do. There are different stations including the shop, the door, the dining room. We make beds, get patients up, give them clothing, take them to the dining room. Then we do our cleaning.

We do everything. They change us around all the stations and an attendant can't say which she likes. I like the pantry.

I like the insulin room less because sometimes the patients give trouble.

One of the aspects of the attendants' role that they seldom mention is the fact that they possess, or they can ask the nurses for, the keys to the dormitories, lockers, store rooms, and even the exits and entrances to the pavilion, a symbol that has great import in a psychiatric hospital (Loeb 1968:306-307) and also gives them a certain power and authority over the patients. Other aspects of the attendant's role were revealed in the responses to the question, 21. "What qualities should a person have for this work?"; and if the question was not understood, the additional question, "Could any person carry out this work?" What the attendants answered reflects not just the expectation of physical labor--although their use of the word "work" appears to have a narrow meaning concretized in "cleaning" and in taking a passive role in the sense of "obeying", or "carrying out orders"--but there is also an active and prideful element in their identity as guardian, which is one part of the role, as well as in their aspirations to learn less passive skills and their deeper feelings, rudimentary as they may be, regarding patients' humanity with, perhaps, a residuum of fear of a strange condition:

> Attendant José Alfaro: We risk our lives. You've seen what happens with patients who are so aggressive. At the time I came here I was something of a boy and I was afraid that some patient would grab me and hit me. When they came near me, I ran away. Later, little by little, I learned to work. I think that just anybody can't work here because, you know, there's a lot of danger. The person who comes here would have to be able to do the work. It would have to be a serious person in good condition, and obedient in service.

> Attendant Carmen Bravo: Any person could carry out the work, for example, in the sense that this is a mental hospital. Well, then not in the case of a person who was afraid to work here. It depends on character or getting used to it. Many people are afraid that something will happen to them.

> Attendant Enrique Costa: His conduct should be good and he should be able to do the work. Any person could do it. [I ask him, "And should he be physically strong?"] Very tough, too. He should also have patience and be pleasant with the patients.

> Attendant Manuel Chacón: Just any person couldn't come here. You've got to have a good background, not a bad one. In the second place you have to be willing to do the work. You need to behave yourself. A person needs a good conduct certificate, blood analysis, and a medical examination to see if he's in condition to work. The resident doctor looks over all the papers you bring. Then he gives you a physical examination. Your body has to be in good condition.

> Attendant Francisco Durán: You have to carry out the work. Just any person can't be hired, because there are many of us who are not in good health. You have to be interested in the work and behave honorably. [I probe on toughness.] You have to be tough, too, but

some patients are weak and you can't act the same way with them as you do with the rest.

Attendant Carlos Estrada: To apply for work a person needs his electoral identification, military identification, good conduct certificate, dispensary certificate, blood certificate, and recommendations from some people, that's all. He has to be big enough so he can keep up with his fellow workers and so he can help the others in pacifying an agitated patient. When a patient comes in you have to let the bosses know, and when somebody calls on the telephone you have to give the message to the nurses.

Attendant Luis Fuentes: You have to be over the age of 20. When there are vacancies, any person older than 20 could work here. Otherwise, it depends on character. You've got to have a lot of patience here for dealing with the patients. When an attendant hits a patient, they fire him. A violent person would get into fights all the time, and a timid person couldn't work here.

Attendant Alberto García: Above all, when you come for the first time, you have to have all your papers, your good conduct certificate, health certificate, venereal certificate. You also have to be healthy and have recommendations. You need to be friendly with the patients, have a good character, respect all of the personnel, your companions as well as your bosses. You have to try to avoid any problem with a patient. There are patients often who come up to you to hurt you. You have to evade it and get out of there.

Attendant Nestor Hoyos: You have to be obedient, respectful, friendly with the patients, and interested in working. Then the nurses will be satisfied. You have to be tough so you can defend yourself, because some patients turn aggressive.

Attendant Pablo Ibáñez: You have to act properly and be patient, especially with the patients, so you can stand them there. At least you shouldn't be violent, and you mustn't irritate them. You have to be attentive whatever they say. Some ask for favors like having a bath or asking the nurse for soap. We help them.

Attendant Tomás Jiménez: You have to know how to deal with patients and get along with the bosses, or at least the doctor. You're at the orders of the doctors and nurses.

Attendant Jorge León: First, you need to have an education, at least to the fourth year of primary school. This is the main thing. You have to be healthy. When you come to apply, you have to come with all your papers. They need to see that a person is going to be useful. You have to be obedient, behave yourself, because how you behave always says a lot. They don't hesitate to fire you. You need to be respectful with the bosses, and with your companions too. You have to know how to deal with the patients.

Attendant Augusto Llona: You just have to be peaceful, but you shouldn't be timid because some of the patients often become aggressive. You should remember that they're suffering from mental illness and they don't know what they're doing.

Attendant Germán Meza: You have to be punctual and get along well with the patients and the bosses. That's it. Some people are too young. Some don't have all their papers in order. If there's a vacancy, any person can come. There are a lot of people who want to work here but there's no vacancy. You have to understand this atmosphere. Then you're not afraid. A lot of people find that this work with mental patients is very difficult because they're dangerous.

Attendant Ana Nores: They need capable and educated people. They're required to have a primary education. A person has to have her papers. If there's a vacancy, and if we're lucky, we're hired. Or if a person can be recommended by the bosses. Any person can be hired. They don't hire women who are too short, but if they have good recommendations, sure, they hire them.

Attendant Luisa Ortiz: You have to know how to get along with the patients. For example, when they need you, you have to give them what they want. You've always got to entertain them. Some of them aren't conscious. That's all.

Attendant Yolanda Paredes: When there are vacancies, you need a medical certificate, educational certificate, and recommendations, that's all. You also have to have the character for this work, in the sense of not being afraid of mental patients.

Attendants' desires to acquire skills are revealed in their responses to questions, 25 and 26. "Have you received any training to perform an attendant's work?"; "Has anyone bothered to train you how to act with patients in a pavilion?" It is noteworthy that with the first question many attendants did not see as "training" various attempts, though lacking in structure, by different resources in the Hospital to give them an orientation to their work, although they clearly recognized these same attempts as "training" in the context of the second question:

> Attendant José Alfaro: One of my comrades told me, "Look, fellow, here are the customs. Bring your broom and clean up here." Then he told me to be very careful with the patients, that some were this way and others were that way. I was thankful, but it seemed very strange to me to be working in this kind of a hospital and looking at the way the patients were. I thought that maybe I wasn't going to be working here, after all. But time passed and now I'm used to it. I got to know the patients and we became friends. I thought at the beginning that I'd never get used to it. I had a cousin from up north who came to work here. He stayed for a month and then he got out. He told me, "If I can't get used to general service, how can you stay in a pavilion?" He was a gardener and worked outside in the park.
>
> Only my comrades trained me how to defend myself when an agitated patient attacked.

> Attendant Enrique Costa: No, none.
>
> Yes, my aunt who was also working here trained me. She told me how to treat the patients and how to act with the bosses.

> Attendant Manuel Chacón: No, none.
>
> Yes, when you get hired the supervisors put you in touch with all the things you need to know to work here, how you need to get along with the patients, get along with superiors, the nurses on the service, and be respectful with everybody, even the patients. They tell you to be good to the patients and take care of them in every way possible.

> Attendant Francisco Durán: Yes, from the nurses, Señorita Arruga and Señorita Frías. They told me practical things for getting the work done and how to get along well with my comrades and with the patients.
>
> Yes, the nurses showed me that I should treat them with the greatest affection.

> Attendant Carlos Estrada: When I was hired, yes, like how a patient should be treated when he's agitated, how to grab him without hitting him when he doesn't want to go to the nurses' station, and how to bring him there for his treatment. If he doesn't want to pay attention to the nurse, you take him by the arm and pull him to where

he has to be. Then they told me that the stations that were assigned to me had to be quite clean. A nurse trained me like that when I came to work.

Yes, the doctors and the nurses, too, warned me that a person who didn't carry out his obligation would be sent to another pavilion. The other day there was an attendant here who didn't do his work properly. He didn't do a good job of cleaning. One of the doctors told the secretary to send him to Pavilion [n]. The nurses always give us advice. Señorita Frías is very good. She always gives good advice.

Attendant Alberto García: When I came to work the nurse told me how patients should be treated, how things were run, what the service was like, and how to help with rounds.

Sure, here with the nurses. They let me know what was happening. They told me what to do. You need to get the bosses' trust. That way you can learn something and work better. The nurses have more education and it's good to get close to them to find out what's going on.

Attendant Nestor Hoyos: Yes, there was an old comrade who taught me what the work was like, what had to be done. That was Estrada. He knew what the work was like. A person who comes in from the street doesn't know these things.

Yes, first that you shouldn't hit them or treat them badly. Then, to feed them, get them dressed, help them go to bed. Then, that they're clean. I learned all that from my comrade Estrada and from the nurse.

Attendant Jorge León: No, you learn by yourself, watching what your comrades are doing. You learn little by little.

Yes, I had a brother who was working here, before, and he let me know what to do with the patients. He knew how to deal with them and get along well with them.

Attendant Ana Nores: Before, Dr. Obregón used to give us classes. He taught us about the patients, how to stop them when they became violent, so they wouldn't hurt us. I don't remember how many classes we had. They haven't had those classes for around 2 years. I don't know why. Most of us have been here for a while. We've all had those classes. They used to have them for 2 hours once a week.

The responses to the question, 27, "Would you like to receive special training?", provide much information, not only about the attendants' condition but also about their aspirations. The reader may take note of the frequency with which attendants mention their desire to learn how to give injections. This may be taken as a highly significant symbol of their desires to acquire a skill, more power over their lives, better incomes, and greater social weight in the Hospital:

> Attendant José Alfaro: I'd like that a lot. It's good to get instruction on how to defend yourself. If you come on the job without that, what happens? It seems to me that there should be someone here to teach you how you should defend yourself. When a comrade is hired he learns from his comrades. A course would leave us a little better off. They also should teach about contagious diseases, how to protect yourself against microbes and to clean your hands.
>
> Attendant Carmen Bravo: Yes, an orientation for new attendants. They should be trained in a short course, or an apprenticeship, where they should be taught how to deal with patients. It should be explained to them the reasons why this should be done and what patients are like.
>
> Attendant Enrique Costa: Of course, to be like a nurse's aide. I'd like to take courses and practice at the same time, all relating to service in the Hospital as a profession.
>
> Attendant Manuel Chacón: Why not? They should teach practice, how to give injections, the things that go on in the Hospital. They ought to give technical courses, too.
>
> Attendant Francisco Durán: Yes, medicine for example.
>
> Attendant Carlos Estrada: Yes, for example, I'd like them to teach me how to give injections. That's all.
>
> Attendant Luis Fuentes: Of course, so as to defend yourself against patients who are aggressive.
>
> Attendant Alberto García: Yes. First, when you're hired, they should teach you what patients are like and how you ought to act with them. When I came to insulin therapy for the first time, the nurses taught me how to get them up, how to feed them breakfast. Every attendant is given his place for watching the patients and seeing that

they and the place are clean. There ought to be a class for nurses' aides, on how to take pulses and give injections.

Attendant Nestor Hoyos: Of course, they should teach us how to give injections in case of an emergency.

Attendant Pablo Ibáñez: Of course. They don't give us anything. There's nobody to do it. You discover things on your own. It would be better like that, but there's none of that. It would be on how to clean a floor, for example, how to clean it better.

Attendant Tomás Jimenez: Yes, for example, to give injections like a practical nurse.

Attendant Jorge León: Of course. I'd like to learn how go give injections. A person wants to learn things beyond cleaning up. We lack a lot of knowledge that could help us in case of emergencies. You can't get trained here because there's no room for it.

Attendant Augusto Llona: Yes. I'd like to receive special training for those of us in insulin, for example, to learn what it is and what has to be done when a patient goes into a coma, because many times when some patient is outside the pavilion he goes into a coma. Then a person could help him so as not to call the nurse.

Attendant Germán Meza: I'm satisfied with what I received, but it would be good to have training in things a person hasn't met with before, like what he has never done. We have talks with the doctors, and I like that a lot. I'd like to have more of them. The doctors talk to us about different diseases and what patients are like. They tell us to let them know that they shouldn't worry, to explain to them that they're not going to be here forever. We just had that for a while and then it stopped. They don't do it now. We were glad. We got together every Wednesday or Thursday to learn about their diseases and how to help them.

Attendant Ana Nores: Yes, I'd like it. I'd like to learn nursing.

Attendant Luisa Ortiz: It would be wonderful if they'd give us that. It would be something to take more advantage of what a person doesn't know. It would be for the patients. A person would like to have them teach how to give injections, take temperatures and pulses. That's all.

Attendant Yolanda Paredes: Of course. Giving injections would be a great thing.

Hospital discipline tends to be strict, as is evident in the responses to many of the questions, and an attendant who has committed offenses against it can be discharged. This is a serious matter in a poor country with a high rate of unemployment. Thus, attendants focus their attention on keeping their jobs and pay less attention to lesser sanctions. It is not surprising that they do not emphasize the Hospital's use of transfer from better to worse pavilions as a type of discipline. This possibility appears more clearly in their responses to questions about their preferences among the pavilions (Appendix to this chapter, questions 16-18), where they express their attraction to clean and less dangerous pavilions, and their repulsion from the dirty ones, those where patients are notorious for being violent, and those reserved for contagious diseases (tuberculosis). Otherwise, the questions which brought out disciplinary matters were, 30, "What are the things that an attendant can not do?" and 31, "How can an attendant be discharged from work? Why? If it is unjust, can one complain? To whom?":

Attendant José Alfaro: The nurse can try to let an attendant know. If the nurse hates him, he can tell him that he's done a bad job or he can send him to another pavilion. An attendant has the right to defend himself. He can go to the supervisors' office to make a complaint. There are things that can seem bad to the nurse. You can do good cleaning and even them not satisfy him. You can't smoke on the service. You can't play cards with patients, although you certainly can do it off the service if you're free. If you don't behave yourself and if you don't apply yourself to your work, you can be suspended or fired from the hospital. For example, you can't fight with patients.

[Response to the second question is reproduced in Chapter 3.]

Attendant Enrique Costa: You can't do treatments and things that are out of your reach. You can't smoke or be doing things contrary to the service.

You can be discharged for offending a patient or a boss. If it's unjust, well, you can complain to the union you belong to.

Attendant Manuel Chacón: [Response to the first question and first part of the second is reproduced in Chapter 3.]

You can go to the supervisors' office to make a complaint. If they don't accept it you can go to the union headquarters and they will present a claim or a petition to the Charity Society. It's been done and attendants have won.

Attendant Carlos Estrada: You can't talk back inside the pavilion or hit patients or let some strange person come in.

For example, someone who refuses to do his work, if he doesn't carry out his obligations, or for a lot of offenses he's committed, or when he takes something out of the pavilion like clothing or some other thing that belongs to the Hospital. They fired an attendant from Pavilion [n] because they discovered him taking out bedsheets. Sometimes they suspend a person for no reason, when another attendant is at fault and they don't find out the truth. This happened to me when I was working in Pavilion [n]. A doctor sent me out to Pavilion [n] without a reason. I was on service. It was in the afternoon when a patient suddenly started to hit the nurse because he didn't want to take his pills. I grabbed him and took him to bed. We fell on the floor and the other patients told the doctor that I'd hit him. The nurse defended me, but it didn't make any difference to the doctor. That's the only thing that happened to me here in the Hospital. In Pavilion [n] an attendant hit a patient with a broom, and the patient told the nurse that another attendant had done it. They should find out first before they punish a person. That attendant didn't protest but they only suspended him. You can make a protest in the supervisors' office. They're paying attention to us now. Not in the past, but we have our association that speaks for us.

Attendant Alberto García: An attendant can't give a patient injections, or take his pulse or his temperature, because all that has to to with nurses' work. There are a lot of attendants who are beligerant, who don't carry out orders from the nurses. An attendant has to be sober. He can't come to work drunk. He has to come in condition for working. If a person is sick, he goes to the resident doctor who gives him time off. If it's serious, the doctor from Workers' Social Security comes to his house to take care of him. If he needs an operation, they take him to the hospital. A person has to let the head of personnel know about it. If he doesn't let them know within three days, they discharge him. A sick attendant gets his whole wage for the first month. They begin to discount in the second month. Then he can return to work with no trouble.

[Response to the second question is reproduced in Chapter 3.]

Attendant Pablo Ibáñez: An attendant can't give injections or do paper work because that's work for the nurse, and an attendant can't intrude on it. He doesn't give medications or answer the telephone, except in an emergency, and even then he can't answer if the nurse is there.

[Response to the second question is reproduced in Chapter 3.]

Attendant Tomás Jiménez: An attendant can't misbehave with the bosses or offend the patients. The bosses are bosses from the administration, doctors and nurses. Mainly, a person shouldn't hit patients because they're mental patients and they don't know what they're doing. The duties are not leaving the service, performing the work assigned, and not leaving the station unless a boss tells him to.

[First part of response to the second question is reproduced in Chapter 3.] They can suspend or discharge. If it's the first time, they suspend a person, but on the second or third he's discharged.

Attendant Jorge León: Comrades can't fight if there's trouble between them. If they fight they're discharged. It's a bad thing.

They discharge a person, also, if he wants to take home some useful thing. I know about a case. He was stealing. It went on for something like four or five years. A gentleman came and fired him. It happened in another pavilion. I also knew a man who was working in the kitchen. He hit a patient there on the spot. The patient was working well and helping the cooks. He did everything but the cook hit him, his own assistant. They fired the man. The patient was peeling potatoes and the cook told him to do something else. The patient didn't want to and disobeyed. Then the cook kicked him and the patient fought back. They fired the cook but they didn't do anything to the patient because it wasn't his fault. An attendant can complain to the Federation, and if the thing isn't serious they get his job back for him. There was a strike in 1956. They stopped work for three hours. It was that cook that they didn't want to take back. But finally they took him. They wouldn't do that in the case of stealing because it's a very bad thing. There have been a few strikes, just stoppages for a few hours, for pay, for the bonus. There was one other time but I don't remember why. The Federation includes all the workers in the Charity Society. We consider ourselves workers. There's another federation for the employees.

Attendant Augusto Llona: For example, you can't apply a syringe. Also, you can't give pills without orders from a nurse. You can't let a patient out without an order. And you can't leave the service.

[First part of response to the second question is reproduced in

Chapter 3.] During the time I've been working here, once there was an attendant who was going out by the side gate [from the Hospital grounds]. The guard put his hand in the attendant's bag. He didn't do it to look for anything but just to try the attendant's patience. And when the attendant got violent the guard reported him and they fired him. They took him to the police station. That shows that you shouldn't be violent. You should tolerate a lot of things. Violence isn't good for us. That's the only case since I've been working here.

Attendant Ana Nores: An attendant can't give injections, take temperatures, or take histories. Those are the job of the nurses.

[Response to the second question is reproduced in Chapter 3.]

Although the attendant does heavy work in the pavilion, and spends more time with patients than any other member of the Hospital's personnel, his or her estimation of himself/herself is low or at least constricted. This is shown in the responses to the question, 38. "What importance does the attendant's work have in the Hospital?" It is to be noted that, when I used the word "empleado" in interviewing in Spanish, my first informant quickly corrected me. In many cases, when the subject did not understand the question, I tried to explore ambiguous responses with another question, "In what sense?":

Attendant José Alfaro: We are workers and the others are public employees. We're not public employees but workers. This is shown on the social security cards. Even the secretary [of this pavilion] is a worker.

Attendant Carmen Bravo: It's very important, for the most part with patients. The attendant looks after the patients. The job is taking care of them, working a lot with the nurses. It's a help for them. What would they do without the attendants?

Attendant Enrique Costaz He has the obligation of looking out for the patients and taking care of them.

Attendant Manuel Chacón: It's important for him to be present to take care of the patients because sometimes they fight. Sometimes they could kill each other.

Attendant Francisco Durán: Yes, he's important. In the sense of helping with the treatments that are given to patients by order of the nurses or the doctors.

Attendant Carlos Estrada: The importance is in watching the patients and doing the cleaning.

Attendant Luis Fuentes: Of course he's important because he's always called on to do the cleaning.

Attendant Alberto García: Performing out his work, carrying out his obligation, collaborating.

Attendant Nestor Hoyos: Yes, he's important because he lends his services.

Attendant Pablo Ibáñez: It's important because it consists in having the service clean and everything in its place.

Attendant Tomás Jiménez: It's carrying out superiors' orders. It's important because that way a person shows the boss what he is, and that he can carry out the job he's been assigned by himself without the bosses having to stay around and watch him.

Attendant Jorge León: Of course it's important. The importance is that we're usually here because of the problems of working outside.

Attendant Augusto Llona: Yes, it's very important. In the first place, for doing service in the station the nurse assigns you, for doing the cleaning, watching the patients, and going on errands for the nurse.

Attendant Germán Meza: If there weren't attendants there'd be a lot of fights, and so a person has to be in control with them all the time.

Attendant Ana Nores: Important? I don't think so, but it's always necessary to have personnel. If there were no personnel the patients would do whatever they wanted, hitting each other and fighting among themselves.

Attendant Luisa Ortiz: Yes, she's important for the nurses. We have the responsibility of taking care of them. If anything happens they suspend us. If they escape and go back home, they suspend us for two or three days.

I asked the attendants if the job had changed (Appendix, question 39.), a bad question because they were unable to answer, and then, a little more productively about the best and worst aspects of their work (Appendix, question 40.), and which aspect was most important (Appendix, question 41.). In general, they responded to question 40. in terms of "carrying out obligations," "earning a living," "it's easy work," "the hours are set," and so on regarding the best aspects; and "you could be attacked" or "you don't make money without working" regarding the worst aspects. To 41., they tended to reply with something like "carrying out obligations." Only Attendant Jorge León gave a non-stereotyped response:

> The advantage it has is that, first, we have social security, because that's indispensable. Second, because we're unionized, and if something happens they protest for you and they put you back to work again. If you need something, you can go to the administration and they give it to you, discounting your wages little by little. They don't just give us money or things, but they give us invoices for things that we need in our houses, a radio, a table, whatever. We get this things discounted. The disadvantages are that they don't give you work clothes, like, for example, in food service when we get dirty. We've asked several times, but they don't want to do it. The Federation asked the administrative assistant. In the Hospital Dos de Mayo, sure, they give clothing. Here they don't want to. It would be an expense of 18 thousand soles, and with one change it would be another 18 thousand. Also the food is on the bad side. We can come in any time to eat, even on our days off. We get the same food, no matter what pavilion we're working in. The food's better with the paying patients, but they only send the necessary food and so the attendants can't take advantage of it. Our food is a little better than what charity patients get. The paying patients get first class food.

Only later questions, 50-51., "What do you do with patients aside from your duties?" and "What would you like to do?", managed to bring out a little more the attendants' ideas about their activities in their pavilions as well as about the possibilities for engaging in more therapeutic activities. Although the responses were short, and also stereotyped, they are worthy of presentation even if they only illustrate the difficulties the attendants had in formulating responses to questions which cut across the grain of their habitual thought processes. However, these responses are also texts that perhaps may be more usefully read for what they do not say than for what they do say about attendants' reactions:

> Attendant José Alfaro: When a person finishes his service? We have to look at them, see that nothing happens to them, see that they're clean and that they don't escape. After lunch, we talk and read the newspapers.
>
> If I'm not busy with my work, I'd like to talk with them, ask them what's in the newspapers, and discuss soccer.
>
> Attendant Carmen Bravo: I've talked with them, played cards and checkers. Other games.
>
> I'd like to see them doing work with their hands, labor therapy. Pavilion [n] has a shop that I saw once. They also do leather work there. We ought to have that here.
>
> Attendant Enrique Costa: I engage in conversation, or play games. Sometimes I take them to the soccer field.
>
> I'd like to talk and play games, like that, the way I said.
>
> Attendant Manuel Chacón: I bring them fruit, soap, anything from outside. I buy things for them.
>
> I like to be good to all of them.
>
> Attendant Francisco Durán: I talk to them and share some ideas I have with them.
>
> Help them when it's necessary.
>
> Attendant Carlos Estrada: Sometimes I bring them DDT when there are invoices to get it, and things like gasoline. I bring their clothing from the laundry.
>
> I like to play soccer. Otherwise, I like to talk about sports.
>
> Attendant Luis Fuentes: Apart from service I'm not here. It's not allowed to play cards with patients.
>
> To talk. It would also be good to play. I can't think of anything else.
>
> Attendant Alberto García: I ask them questions, like about how they lived before at home, if they have families, their education. I ask them if they're ill. Most of them say no. Then I ask what they want to do when they get out. I give them advice on how to behave themselves when they're out, and how to behave when they go off to

work.

I'd like to distract them a little, talk with the ones that are isolated, try to reunite them with the rest of their comrades. It's necessary to distract them because they're thinking about a single thing.

Attendant Nestor Hoyos: Games. I make jokes to distract them. Talk to them.

Attendant Pablo Ibáñez: I can't answer.

Talk to them, ask them questions. Sometimes they ask us, or they tell us about their lives, their childhood, their occupations.

Attendant Tomás Jiménez: I start talking about things, but we shouldn't make those patients disturbed.

Show them, for example, how they ought to act with the doctors, with the attendants.

Attendant Jorge León: I don't do anything after I'm finished with work. I go out to the park to rest during my time off.

We'd like to play soccer, if there were a ball.

Attendant Augusto Llona: When we're off service, if we meet some patient outside the pavilion we tell the attendant who is on service so he'll bring him back to the pavilion.

I'd like to take them to the soccer field and watch them play, of course, if they're lucid.

Attendant Germán Meza: Nothing. I just deal with those who are healthy. I try to talk with them, have some conversations.

I'd like to distract them with games, get their attention in a card game, as we always do when work is over.

Attendant Ana Nores: Nothing. [She laughs.]

If they'd ask me some favor, I'd cooperate. Maybe some purchase outside.

Attendant Luisa Ortiz: We bring them things they need.

We're going to sew because we have labor therapy here.

Attendant Yolanda Paredes did not answer.

The attendants appeared cautious in answering the questions (Appendix, questions 42-44.) about doctors, ones which dealt with how they were, how they ought to be, how they treated the attendants, and which was the best. There was little variation in the responses: "They're good," "They treat us well," "They are considerate to us," "They're good people," "They ought to know how to get along with attendants," "They have to look after the patients," "They should show kindness and trust to inferiors," "I don't know them." Most were willing to name "the best doctor," but almost all of them qualified their statements, saying that "the others are also good."

Most of them responded in the same way in regard to nurses (Appendix, questions 45-47.): "They're good people," "They're friendly," "They're the same to me," "Some are good and others are a little bad," "They ought to get along with an attendant," "They ought to get along with everybody," "I like them all," "I can't say that I like one more and another less," and so on.

As for the patients, attendants had their very specific likes and dislikes. Their responses to the items (Appendix, questions 48-49.) on the individuals they liked most and least show that attendants favor obedient patients, less aggressive ones, the clean, the courteous, those who help them in their tasks, those with whom they can converse; and they disfavor the aggressive, those who escape, those who say dirty things, those who dirty up the pavilion, and the disturbed ones.

Although a psychiatric hospital is not the only place in the world where violence exists, it has the reputation of being a very violent place. Violence occurs and there are few attendants who do not report that they have been the recipients of large and small attacks by patients.[5] It would appear that this is a daily concern for them. They responded to question 33, "Are you at all concerned about the possibilities of harm to your person?":

> Attendant José Alfaro: There's no help. You can do everything they tell you, but there's no help for an attendant because he's poor. You're partly in danger. Maybe something can happen tomorrow. You have to think about that. You have to defend yourself. What are the patients going to do to us?

> Attendant Enrique Costa: Sometimes I worry when I see agitated patients. Sometimes they want to injure an attendant. I'm not worried a lot.

> Attendant Manuel Chacón: Yes, but surely it's according to cases. I'm worried when something happens and then I forget between one

time and another.

Attendant Francisco Durán: Yes, I'm quite worried.

Attendant Nestor Hoyos: Of course, but not much because it's not a disease that attendants can catch.

Attendant Pablo Ibáñez: I worry a little. Sometimes you aren't secure. If you're a little careless you can be attacked in a weak spot. If you're weak. There's an attendant in Pavilion [n] who was attacked by a patient while he was washing his hands. The patient slashed him with a razor. He cut his cheek open from his mouth to his ear. That was about 2 years ago.

Attendant Tomás Jiménez: Yes, but not much. I'm worried when I'm sick or when I'm not in condition to do some thing.

Attendant Jorge León: No, I'm not aware of any harm they can do me, because I don't give any reason to my comrades or to the patients. I get along well with everybody in general. I don't think anybody can do me any harm.

Attendant Germán Meza: Yes, occasionally, because there are a lot of people with different diseases. Many patients have tuberculosis. There's a lot to worry about, but with luck and changing work you bear everything. The attacks by patients are a little different because they happen to everybody. They've put their hands on me, but most of them are smooth.

Attendant Ana Nores: Yes, I'm always worried because there are patients who suddenly attack you. There are violent moments.

Attendant Luisa Ortiz: Yes, because you aren't free and some patients can have at you. It's work that's a danger to your life. I don't worry much but once in a while when patients are disturbed.

Attendant Yolanda Paredes: From the patients? No, I'm not worried. There are times when they want to hit us, but we have to defend ourselves. They go against you, sometimes, when you're taking them to eat. I was bitten on the arm once. [She shows me the scar.]

Thus, many of the attendants see their work as somewhat threatening, although most of them appear to have lost their initial fear. Their experience is reflected in their responses to the questions, 62, "What happened to you when you came to the Hospital to work the first time? How did you feel?," and 63-64, "What things do you consider most important for getting used to it?" and "What were your greatest difficulties?":

Attendant José Alfaro: I was afraid. I couldn't touch a patient.
I got used to it, but I'd rather be a mechanic so as to make enough money.

Attendant Carmen Bravo: I was afraid, distrustful when I came.

Attendant Enrique Costa: When I came on the first day, things seemed very strange and I had to ask questions so the nurse on duty, Señorita Frías, would give me a little orientation about the work. She showed me the way to work.
You have to have a noble character and know how to deal with the patients.
The greatest difficulty is contagion.

Attendant Manuel Chacón: I felt somewhat overwhelmed. I was worried that I could also catch some of that. But it's nothing.
You have to forget your worries about contagion a little and be a little at peace.
The greatest difficulty is contagion.

Attendant Francisco Durán: I felt calm.
I had no difficulty.

Attendant Carlos Estrada: Sure, a little bit afraid for about 5 days, afraid that they'd hit me or kill me. When you come for the first time, it's quite fierce, but you get used to it.
You have to obey the nurse and the doctors.

Attendant Luis Fuentes: It just seemed to me like making work into sport. I felt a little anxious because I'd never worked in a hospital like this one. I was afraid at the beginning. But as I worked, this timidity went away. I got used to it.
You have to get accustomed to the atmosphere.
I don't think I had any.

Attendant Alberto García: I was impressed. I was a little fearful of the patients because I really looked and I saw each one as different. You never see this outside. You watch the patients and get to know them little by little, so you lose that fear.

Above all, you have to have serenity. You have to accept the way the bosses are, and your comrades in work, so that they'll teach you how to act and how to work in a hospital.

Attendant Nestor Hoyos: I felt very strange at the way work was done, because I was a stranger to all my comrades, and at the difference, because outside there's another way of working, first because the work of cleaning is for women [sic]. I was afraid the patients were going to hurt me. After two or three days I lost that.

You're at ease from the way the nurses treat you and from the work which is very easy to do. Sometimes the nurse isn't satisfied with your work or because you've come a little late, and then you're suspended.

The difficulty was because I didn't know a single one of the attendants, or their character. Some are very rude and don't have the kindness to tell a person how things are, or they give bad answers.

Attendant Pablo Ibáñez: When I started I felt quite satisfied to have steady and secure work.

You should be obedient, not talk back to the bosses, and do what they say.

Attendant Tomás Jiménez: I was a little afraid when I was close to a patient who was agitated, but as time passed I got used to it. I got to know the habits of patients and the way to deal with them.

Mainly, you have to be at peace and find yourself in condition to work in a hospital with mental patients.

It was at the beginning when I hadn't got used to the habits and actions of the patients.

Attendant Jorge León: I felt very happy at the fact that I finally had work. I wasn't afraid because I knew how it was from my brother and other friends. Some people are afraid and have to get used to it. Not me.

You need to know people. You have to have friends, and through them you get used to it faster. You learn your job from them.

I didn't have any difficulty.

Attendant Augusto Llona: I felt a little cowardly for not knowing the characteristics of the Hospital, I used to think that maybe some patient was going to hurt me in some way. I didn't have any idea about the precautions that you need to take. When I had worked for a month I was into their atmosphere and then I was easy with them, and with some of them I even had confidence. With taking them out to walk and to the movies, then I felt easy.

You have to be peaceful in this Hospital. You shouldn't be timid or think that some patient's going to hurt you. And you need to be friends with the rest of the attendants and the nurses.

I didn't have any difficulty.

Attendant Germán Meza: I felt a little strange because, in the first place, I was looking at many of them showing a great deal of difference from normal people, the way they acted, their conversation, their smiles, and the movements they made for no reason.

In the first place, you should have work clothes, a work uniform. There ought to be a regular dining room. Above all, food and wages that agree with people because they're enough.

Attendant Ana Nores: It bothered me. I was afraid when I saw so many patients. Little by little I got used to it. I stayed in view of my need to work. At the beginning I had urges to stop working, because I was repelled when I looked at the patients because I'd never seen such things, like the way they froth at the mouth during treatment, and when I saw electroshock.

An attendant should have force of will, in view of the necessity she has to work.

For me there were moments that bothered me because I didn't understand. I've never liked seeing disgusting things.

Attendant Luisa Ortiz: Since I already knew how to deal with mental patients in X_____ Clinic, it didn't seem strange to me to be with them. It seemed weird there because I'd never dealt with them.

You need character. It's the only thing.

They were that I thought I wouldn't get used to it. All my ideas were what they say outside, that crazy patients hit you, that they're dangerous.

Attendant Yolanda Paredes: I felt unaccustomed. I wanted to go back outside. Then I got used to it. At the beginning it seemed strange to me.

I got used to it after a month. You get used to it as you work for a few years.

To end the interview, I asked the question, 65, "Suppose I were a new attendant who had just come on the job, what advice would you give me for getting used to it faster?" They answered as follows:

> Attendant José Alfaro: Above all, I'd tell you that we're all brothers here in this work and the duties aren't hard. Your life won't end here. In a few days you're going to be fine and you're going to learn what you need to know so you'll get along.
>
> Attendant Carmen Bravo: First, not to mistrust the patients, but I'd tell you which ones you can have confidence in and also the ones with whom you need to be cautious, those who can harm you. I'd put you in contact with them so that you wouldn't worry about them, because when a person comes for the first time, because he or she has been outside and has never been in one of these hospitals, he or she has the idea that these patients are dangerous. But this idea is false. Then, with the personnel, you need to understand each other and get along. And you need to have respect and be obedient with the nurses and doctors.
>
> Attendant Enrique Costa: I'd tell you the way to work, how to deal with the patients, and everything related to the work.
>
> Attendant Manuel Chacón: I'd teach you the customs that have to do with the work, and also all the characteristics that each one of them has, and I'd try to lift your spirits so you wouldn't feel discouraged, so that your spirit wouldn't react by getting lower.
>
> Attendant Francisco Durán: I'd tell you to look for friends among the older attendants and the head of personnel.
>
> Attendant Carlos Estrada: I'd teach you the work, how it is. Then the way to deal with the patients, not to hit them, and to pay attention to the nurse and carry out the work.
>
> Attendant Luis Fuentes: I'd tell you to take precautions, not to be timid. Nothing else, I think.
>
> Attendant Alberto García: Above all, to try to make yourself a comrade, to make friends and have confidence. I'd let you know what the treatment is like, show you how to clean and how to keep the service in good condition, and how to avoid arguments with the nurse or the doctor. I'd advise you how you should try to avoid

patients who are misbehaving.

Attendant Nestor Hoyos: I'd be friendly with you and show you how to do things, how to act with the nurse, his moods, and which comrades are good and in whom you can have confidence. I'd tell you that the doctor comes for his work hour, and then that you can't say anything to the nurse. I'd go with you to eat, and always show you how things are done. Then we'd be friends.

Attendant Pablo Ibáñez: I'd teach you how we act here. After that, a person can get used to it. The advice would be not to be afraid of the patients, because some new attendants are afraid. I'd tell you to behave yourself with the bosses and the comrades, what has to be done, what happens at certain times. The others taught me that and I got used to it quickly.

Attendant Tomás Jiménez: Mostly, I'd tell you about all the customs that have to do with working, and I'd try to convince you that in time you're going to get used to the way things are done and the way the bosses and the patients treat you. Because working in a hospital with mental patients, a person ought to do the best he can during work.

Attendant Jorge León: I'd tell you to act right, respect the bosses, and obey what they order, to have consideration for them and get along well with them, and to know how to deal with patients. Also to be on time to work and not to be absent.

Attendant Augusto Llona: It would be to have a little distrust in the patients. I'd give you all the details about them, those who are aggressive and other lucid ones, so that in this way you can work peacefully, always taking care with certain ones. I'd teach you to make up your service, and show you the whole pavilion so you'd know where clothes storage was, the whole service, and the cleaning equipment. I'd tell you to respect the nurses and obey them in everything, and also to try to have more confidence in all the other attendants so that, in this way, you'll be easy and without any kind of worries that exist outside, and that you put your whole attention into your work.

Attendant Germán Meza: In the first place, I'd give you an idea about the work and what the customs are like. In the second place, I'd teach you about how to act toward people to whom you owe respect. Also, according to what you're doing, about the character of things, about the way of showing up at the correct time, both coming in and leaving. And then how you start the work that you need to do. That would be everything.

Attendant Ana Nores: That you needn't pay attention, that you should ignore everything that happens, and always protect yourself from the patients who can hurt you. I'd teach you how to clean the service, that it's not good to get friendly with anyone without knowing her. I'd make you aware of what they're saying. There are plenty of people who talk hypocritically. I'd tell you about the boss and how to get along with her.

Attendant Luisa Ortiz: I'd teach you how to deal with a patient, how to take care of her, what the service is like, and how you need to be, and how to entertain a patient so she won't be sad. That's all.

Attendant Yolanda Paredes: I'd teach you how things should be done, how you should act. That is always taught to a new comrade when she's just come.

Conclusion

Many people who enter a psychiatric hospital for the first time experience a sense of danger and also a sensation of being in a strange and mysterious place. This is clear in the statements of the attendants who have made the transition from an uncertain and anxious beginning, conditioned by the popular idea that such a hospital is a "lunatic asylum," a strange and dangerous place, to an acceptance of his or her work as an ordinary and a daily activity.[6] In other words, an impossible labor becomes performable. More than that, a reading of these texts reveals that in Peru many of the attendants feel that they are fortunate to have steady work in an insecure world where much unemployment, poverty, and need exist. Thus, not only does the strange become ordinary but misfortune becomes good luck. And madness becomes a thing instead of a reflection: as Foucault (1965:70) suggests, the life of the non-patient in an asylum is manageable because madness is externalized and becomes "a thing to look at" while it ceases to be "a monster inside oneself."

A deeper understanding of the fear of madness may be gained by reference to an essay by Freud (1955a), written in 1919, on "The Uncanny," which carries out very skillfully the task of deconstructing the German words *heimlich*, pertaining to the home or the familiar, and *unheimlich*, opposed to the familiar, the strange, or that which causes fear. Freud (ibid.:234, 236, 241, 243) indicates that the uncanny is related to themes of the double, "the repetition of the same features or character-traits or vicissitudes, of the same crimes, or even the same names," but what gives the double the quality of the uncanny is that it comes "from the fact of the 'double' being a creation dating back to a very early mental state, long since surmounted," which "has become a thing of terror, . . . the gods turned into demons." What is frightening is that "every affect belonging to an emotional impulse, whatever its kind, is transformed, if it is repressed, into anxiety, [so that] among instances of frightening things there must be one class in which the frightening element can be shown to be something repressed which *recurs*." In the case of madness a person sees "the working of forces hitherto unsuspected in his fellow-men, but at the same time he is dimly aware of them in remote corners of his own being." Freud (ibid.:248-249, 252) suggests that if through reality testing "repressed infantile complexes," e.g., castration, womb fantasies, and so on, are conquered instead of repressed fears of the uncanny disappear, although he concludes that "the majority of human beings have never become quite free."

If this last point that Freud makes applies to the cases which have been explored here, we may appropriately conclude that the texts presented hide more than they reveal of the conscious and unconscious fears of their authors. If a person who has some insight prefers not to expose his or her conscious fears in such a way as to project a timid presence, such a person's unconscious processes are buried too deep for exposure in a superficial interview. But it is not our task to expose what people prefer to keep hidden; moreover, it is obvious that the attendants are used to the environment of a psychiatric hospital--and those who have not been able to adapt have withdrawn from the situation--, and to the features of mental illness and psychiatric patients, who could be their doubles, their reflections in the pavilion-mirror, reflections in reverse, two-dimensional reflections, reflections of the beginning and the end of the world, reflections of their sins and their innocences. But now they can get along in this environment, perhaps with regressions to more primary states from time to time; and they could be therapeutic resources in the Hospital. That they do not recognize themselves as such is due to the manner in which they and others define their role. Surely their desires to know something, to do more than cleaning, to acquire skills, and *their very clearly stated conceptions of themselves as helpers of patients*, offer great advantages to administrative psychiatry.

Strauss, et al. (1964:118-119), in their research on two North American psychiatric hospitals, found that attendants did indeed organize activities for patients, although these activities were introduced not to give therapy but to "help" patients because they were not the same as the professional "therapeutic" programs. It would appear that a similar aspect of the manner in which Peruvian attendants function is not lacking. Still, Greenblatt (1955:64-65) contemplates even more for the future attendant:

> Bringing attendants into membership in this team implies, first, that they be accepted as individuals; that the fears, tensions, and frustrations facing them in the performance of their jobs be recognized and handled; that steps be taken to improve their skill in dealing with the sick persons who present inexplicable behavior; and that they be given access to sources of information that help to guide the physician in his elaborate considerations of the welfare of the patient. A goal imposed upon the attendant that carries the expectation of additional work and responsibility without increased recognition is not likely to be reached.

Hyde (1955:76-77) amplifies these concepts:

> Once attendants regard themselves as active members of the treatment team and appreciate their interactions with patients as either valuable or hurtful to the latter, then they become not just caretakers of the ward but rather therapists who must grow day by day, month by month, in their understanding, until as time goes by they arrive at those skills which can be expected to bring about favorable changes in a patient's behavior. This ability to create changes rests upon a deep understanding of both the patients and themselves. Without an understanding of themselves it is impossible for personnel to realize what impulses the patients in turn arouse in them.

Thus, it seems clear that there exist possibilities for the utilization of Peruvian attendants in roles that go far beyond those that they enact in the contemporary Hospital. But would it be justice to train attendants, give them skills, without adequate remuneration? Salisbury (1962:122) says in his discussion of a situation in which attendants were educated to the point where "they accepted the same goals as the therapists":

> If such an education were successful, and attendants became as oriented to "curing" as the therapists are, it would in fact make the "therapeutic community" a reality. Some practical difficulties suggest themselves, however, For the attendants, the satisfaction of feeling that they were doing a humanitarian job would have to compensate for the strain involved in the tense and tedious everyday ward situation. Attendants of a different caliber and personality would be required. They would probably consider themselves as professionally trained personnel, yet would still be needed to count blankets or change the clothing of incontinent patients. Their pay scales would also need revision, if such people were to be recruited.

If the escalation of health costs is a serious problem in developed countries, it is out of consideration for underdeveloped ones. Politico-economic questions enter discussion at this point and so it appears that the possibilities of the transformation we have been discussing are excluded, pending resolutions of the struggle for the social distribution of the collective product and the problematic of a State directed by individuals from elite social sectors, who lack the most remote understanding of the roots of their own impulses to retain their personal property and perpetuate the existing social order. In contrast with hospital attendants in developed countries, where the paraprofessional movement has gone much farther, the Peruvian attendants will have to defer their hopes.

Appendix: The List of Questions

1. Name, age, date.
2. Place of birth. Years in Lima
3. Education.
4. Occupations before finding work in the Hospital. Time in each one.
5. Why did you look for work as an attendant in this Hospital?

6. How did you get this work?
7. What do your relatives, your friends, think about your job here?
8. How long have you worked as an attendant here? Other hospitals or clinics?
9. Your wages here?
10. Do you also work outside? What work? Income?
11. Are you married? Children?
12. Is your income enough?
13. How much longer do you expect to continue work here?
14. What would you like to do to earn a living?
15. How is the job of attendant here in general?
16. In which pavilions have you worked?
17. Which do you prefer and why?
18. Which do you dislike and why?
19. What shifts have you worked and which do you prefer?
20. Who contracted you to work here?
21. What qualities should a person have for this work? Could any person carry out this work?
22. What are the attendant's duties (or tasks)?
23. Which do you like most?
24. Which do you like least?
25. Have you received any training to perform an attendant's work?
26. Has anyone bothered to train you how to act with patients in a pavilion?
27. Would you like to receive special training?
28. Who directs the attendant to do his work?
29. Who directs the pavilions?
30. What are the things that an attendant can not do?
31. How can an attendant be discharged from work? Why? If it is unjust, can one complain? To whom?*
32. If a disturbed patient damages your clothing, do you get new clothing?
33. Are you at all concerned about the possibilities of harm to your person? Have you ever been attacked?*
34. How do you get a patient up who does not want to get up?*
35. How do you get a patient to eat who does not want to eat*
36. What do you do when a disturbed patient grabs you?*
37. Should the attendant use force on the patients?*
38. What importance does the attendant's work have in the Hospital?**
39. Has the job of attendant changed?*
40. What is the best aspect of the job? The worst aspect?
41. What is the most important aspect?
42. How are the doctors? How do they treat you?**
43. How should the doctor be?**
44. Who is the best doctor in the pavilion?
45. How are the nurses? How do they treat you?**

46. How should the nurse be?**
47. Whom do you like most? Least?**
48. What type of patient do you like most and why? Whom do you like in this pavilion?
49. What type of patient do you like least and why? Whom in this pavilion?
50. What do you do with patients aside from your duties?
51. What would you like to do?
52. What is the patient's greatest duty?**
53. What thing should Pavilion [n] achieve? What is the goal, why does it exist?*
54. Do you think it is achieving it? How does it do it, or how should it do it?
55. What thing should the Hospital Víctor Larco Herrera achieve? What is the goal, why does it exist?
56. Do you think it is achieving it? How does it do it, or how should it do it?
57. If you could change something in Pavilion [n], what thing or things would it be?
58. What is a mental illness? How does it happen? From where does it come?***
59. Have your ideas changed after working here?
60. What is a hospital like Víctor Larco Herrera?*
61. Have your ideas changed after working here?
62. What happened to you when you came to the Hospital to work the first time? How did you feel?
63. What things do you consider most important for getting used to it?
64. What were your greatest difficulties in getting used to it?
65. Suppose I were a new attendant who had just come on the job, what advice would you give me so I'd get used to it faster?

* Some of the responses to these questions are to be found in Chapter 3.
** Some of the responses to these questions are to be found in Chapter 5.
*** The responses to this question are to be found in Chapter 2.

Notes

1. *Obreros*, workers, and *empleados*, employees, are distinguished according to the two systems of Peruvian social security. Each of these has its own separate bureaucracy, budget, and physical plant, including a hospital. It may be noted that since self-employed workers are not included in any social security system, almost the whole of the peasantry in the rural sector, and the vast "informal" urban sector, are excluded from benefits, which makes the "empleados" of the Hospital Victor Larco Herrera members of a labor elite. Their Hospital wages, together with their supplementary earnings from other

employments, in 1959 placed them in the upper quartile of Peruvian income earners (see Webb 1977:5-17).

2. The complete list of questions is presented in an Appendix.

3. Identities of individuals and places are disguised to protect the privacy of subjects who were kind enough to furnish me with data. The same scheme of alphabetization according to the order of the interviews is employed. I give the attendants first names in this Chapter, since it may be useful to the reader to be able to distinguish gender.

4. In 1959 insulin coma or shock therapy was still in use in Peru. According to James (1992:221, 230-231), in the 1930's it "was initiated without any firm scientific basis, eagerly taken up by psychiatrists worldwide, only to be discarded some twenty years later." He continues, "In the 1950's insulin therapy was increasingly questioned," when controlled studies questioned its effectiveness. Consequently, it "gradually dropped out of use and from standard psychiatric textbooks. . . . In all probability the difficulty in arranging and staffing special units, the hazards of insulin and the greater safety and convenience of oral neuroleptics were additional reasons for the demise of insulin therapy."

5. See Chapter 3 for reports by Attendants Estrada, García, Jiménez, León, Meza, Nores and Ortiz about some of their experiences. I use here only those responses which are not included in that earlier discussion.

6. I have a certain inner familiarity with this transition, having experienced a similar shift from denial to acceptance of madness a half century ago when a member of my family was declared "incompetent" by a judge and locked up in the local mental hospital. I experienced a parallel transition from fear to familiarity in my work in the Hospital Víctor Larco Herrera.

Chapter 7

Mistaken Identities: The Psychiatric Nurses.

The object of this last chapter is to present data about the nurses in the Hospital, taken from the interviews I conducted with them, which will provide an idea of their condition and prospects in 1959. I begin with some general information about nurses in the Hospital, the circumstances of my interviews with them, and their professional situation.

According to information provided by the Hospital's administration, on December 4, 1959 there was a total of 82 graduate nurses working in the Hospital's pavilions. All were graduates of the Hospital's Nursing School, which was the only instructional site for psychiatric nurses in the country. I had the worst success in soliciting interviews with them than with any other category of the Hospital population. The doctors, although they were very busy, were willing to find time to talk with me, and they spoke with enthusiasm about the events of their careers in psychiatry. The attendants were rather pleased to rest for a while during their shifts, and after some initial reserve in most interviews they seemed to feel no great resistance to the relation of information about their life and work. Many of the lucid patients spoke eagerly about their experiences in the pavilion. It was not like that with the nurses. In November and December of 1959, I found only eight nurses who were willing, and had time, to answer my questions. As a supplement to these eight basic interviews, a social worker obtained four more interviews between August and October of 1960.[1] This meager representation is surely due to the fact that they were very busy with their duties during their shifts in the Hospital and--since many of them worked other shifts in other hospitals and clinics, and with private patients outside the Hospital--very busy in their outside shifts, as well. Moreover, and this needs saying, it appears that the ambiguous situation of the nurse, who is the physician's assistant, pavilion administrator, and attendant's "boss" ["*jefe*"], whose identity is thereby fluctuating, provides a structure, and at the same time a lack of structure, which may have led potential interview subjects to keep silent instead of speaking with me. This silence will not have been something simple, but, rather, something very complex. Foucault (1990:27) says:

> Silence itself--the things one declines to say, or is forbidden to name, the discretion that is required between different speakers--is less the absolute limit of discourse, the other side from which it is separated by a strict boundary, than an element that functions alongside the things said, with them and in relation to them within over-all strategies. There is no binary division to be made between what one says and what one does not say; we must try to determine the different ways of not saying such things, how those who can and those who cannot speak of them are distributed, which type of discourse is authorized, or which form of discretion is required in either case. There is not one but many silences, and they are an integral part of the strategies that underlie and permeate discourses.

In the interviews, too, if there are silences in the nurses' responses to my questions, in place of capitulating in the face of the impossibility of making contact with the totality of their reality, we can take our investigation in the direction of the structure in which they exist and function.

To begin, while all nurses recognize their primary duty of giving care to patients, one source of ambiguity is to be found in their linkage to the Hospital, because the nurses' institutional alignment and its consequences should be recognized and stated. According to Osborne (1973:41-42):

> The nurse's primary responsibility is to the institution, since the institution, not the individual patient, employs the nurse, a large component of the nurse's responsibility becomes guiding patients in their adjustment to the requirements of the institution. At times of conflict between patients' needs and institutional requirements, the nurse's choice of loyalty is often biased by her historical, psychological, social, cultural, and economic attachment to the institution.

The nurses of the Hospital Víctor Larco Herrera indeed recognize their ties to the Nursing Supervisors' Office (*Superintendencia*). But now another ambiguity appears in their relations with physicians. I asked only two of the subjects the question, 28.[2] "Who gives orders to the nurse?" Nurse Marta Arruga[3] said: "The doctor. We have the Nursing Supervisors' Office in the Hospital which orders us to different services, but in a pavilion it's the doctor." And Nurse Fernando Bustos reiterated: "The doctor, although they tell you in School [i.e., the Nursing School] that you're independent. In reality the doctor is the director and we have to do what he says. Work is given out in the Nursing Supervisors' Office. They have charge of the attendants and night guards, too." Of course, two responses do not lead to a definitive conclusion with regard to lines of authority, but it appears that while immediate control of nurses in the pavilions lies in the hands of the physicians, the existence of the Nursing Supervisors' Office places nurses in the situation which Henry (1954:141) has called "multiple subordination."

However, the simple subordination of the pavilion-locality, that is, the dependence of the nurse on the physician structures (or destructures?) another vector of ambiguity. Olesen and Whittaker (1968:79) speak of the "traditional subjugation of nursing to its more powerful and male partner, medicine." Glaser (1966:27) says that "nursing . . . works in hospitals run by doctors, that it is bound to obey medical orders for the patient's welfare, and that it is a female and less prestigious occupation confronting a male and more respected one. Doctors have long been accustomed to delegating their routine technical and administrative tasks to nursing service in order to economize on their time."[4] In hospitals there developed a traditional division of labor, which is described by Bellaby and Oribabor (1980:163-164) in their historical exploration of nursing history:

> While medicine sought to "cure", nursing emphasized hygiene and sanitation, and discipline on the ward. But the subsequent proliferation and expansion of hospitals favoured the institutionalization of medicine's curative model. . . .
>
> [The structure of nursing] reproduced in the relation between doctors and nurses the role division between husband and wife, father and mother, in the bourgeois family. Just as the home was the province of women, so the hospital ward was the province of "nurse-housekeepers". . . .
>
> Medical specialization brought in its train the proliferation of ancillary skills: the pharmacist, the X-ray technician and so on. Medicine subordinated these skills. Nurses who were already working under medical direction, became another ancillary skill or rather a group of skills . . . . Further, as medical mastery of technique grew, so several methods, hitherto considered exclusively medical, were handed down to nurses and other ancillary skills as "routine".

Now let us have a look at the interviewed subjects. As was done with the attendants, this presentation of data on the nurses will begin with summaries of the initial questions in the schedule of 56,[5] in order, thus, to give a set of personal pictures of the subjects, their economic, family, and professional situations. Nurses were relatively well off, by Peruvian standards. Except for those who were making current sacrifices in order to continue their education toward other professional careers, the average family income of those who were working double shifts placed them well within the highest 5 percent of Peruvian income earners (see Webb 1977:5-17). Here is what they told me:

> Nurse Marta Arruga: She is 29 years old. She was born in Ch_____, a city on the South Coast. She had nine years of primary and secondary education in Ch_____. She did not finish high school because, although now the requirement for admission to the Nursing School is the complete secondary education of five years, in those times "we could get in with four years of high school." Before she came to school here, she was "nothing but a student." She has been in Lima for fifteen years.
>
> She has worked in this Hospital for eight years. She says: "I came here because I always wanted to be a nurse. Some of my mother's friends were nurses. They came from this School but they were working in Ch_____. I was thinking about [the nursing school in the Hospital] Loayza because the nuns in my high school were from the same order and advised me to go there, but I came directly here

through my mother's friends. I left here for two years to work in the general hospital in Ch_____, and then one day Señorita Alicia [a Supervisor] came to visit and she told me there was an opening here. It was advantagious to work here. I wanted this job and I also wanted to be in Lima. I like this Hospital. I worked in both kinds and I chose this one.

"I also worked in the psychiatric service of the Empleado Social Security [Hospital] for five months, just that. It was last year, in November. I had vacation and leave."

Her salary in this Hospital is 1300 soles a month. Yes, she has another job "in a private home, with one of Dr. Roberto Paz's patients. I work five or six hours a day. When I stay longer it's 5000 soles, and otherwise it's 4000 a month." The income is enough: "I also help my family. I'm working to help them."

She is single, but "I'm planning to get married later."

Nurse Fernando Bustos: He is 26 years old. He was born in a small city on the South Coast. He had his primary education in his home District and high school in the Departmental capital. He has been in Lima for six years. He came directly from home. Before, "I worked in a bank, for just a year, after I graduated from high school."

He worked here as a student nurse for three years and then as a graduate nurse for three more years. He says: "There were three of us who got out of the School and applied to the Supervisors here. There were some vacancies and so we got our jobs in two weeks. There were eighteen girls [sic] and four men in our graduating class. One of the men got a job out of Lima. Three men and one woman [sic] applied here and we got the jobs. We're still working here.

"This Hospital is one of the few where men are working. In those days it was about the only one, because construction of the Empleado wasn't finished yet. Men are working here, in the Empleado, and in public health-aid posts. They give a lot of preference to female personnel. This School and the one in the Police Hospital take men. I don't know about the Military Hospital. The nursing school in the Empleado doesn't take men, just woman."

He earns 1250 soles monthly, with a bonus of 250. He says, "Yes, my income is more or less enough. I'm paying for my education and my brother's. The ones who work outside earn up to 3300. They work in the Hospital del Empleado, but they have to be working fourteen or fifteen hours." He has not been working outside because he has been studying engineering. He says, "Now I'm studying something that I've always liked. I go to the School of Engineering in the National University of Engineering. This is my first year and

I'm in pre-engineering. It's a six-year course.

"I finish here at 1 p.m. Then I study till from 2 to 4:30, and then I attend classes till 8:30. After that, I come back and study till 11. The University is in Rímac [in the eastern part of Lima; the Hospital is located in the extreme west, near the ocean]. It takes about fifty minutes to get there. I read on the bus. It's hard to get an education here in Peru. It's expensive, and engineering is very much so.

"I'm single, not engaged. There's no time."

Nurse Santiago Cruz: He is 28 years old. He was born in a small city in the Central Highlands and had his primary schooling there. He went to the Departmental capital for high school. He finished high school in 1952 and came to Lima in 1953 for further education: "I came to go into the Police School. I didn't get in because it was a matter of influence. So then I went to work as a clerk in a commercial business. It was a store and I waited on customers. I worked there for three years. Then I came to apply to the School in this Hospital, from where I graduated last year.

"This School is the only coeducational school. I had a friend who was working here. He doesn't work here now because he's studying for the priesthood. He got a grant. He's the one who pointed me toward the advantages here. So I took the examinations and put in my papers for entrance.

"I've been working here for eight months. I finished the final examinations in February. They were examinations by the Ministry of Public Health which are given to all the students. I had a month off and then they appointed me to work here. I've never worked elsewhere.

"I earn about 1500 a month with the bonus. They discount it, 2 1/2% for social security, 6% for the union. I don't understand it myself. If you work for thirty years you still get the same salary. I'm learning about all that because I've just started. I don't have any other work for the time being. I'm thinking about it, if not in a hospital then in some public aid post, or on my own account. I haven't made arrangements yet. I went to the public aid post in Miraflores and they told me that when there was a vacancy they'd let me know.

"There's no demand for a private male nurse. Maybe it's because when people are sick they ask more for female nurses. The Empleado is full. It's about the same with the military hospitals [one for each branch of service, plus the police].

"In the afternoons I look over the books I have, physics, chemistry, geometry, because I like to remember all that. Sometimes I play soccer or I visit my parents, because you can't live just for one thing. I have my room in Pavilion 6 where the male nurses live. There are five or six of us, just the bachelors.

"I'm single, still not engaged. The salary isn't enough, not even for a bachelor. You need to go to work in other places."

Nurse Ricardo Chivas: He is 35 years old. He was born in a city in the Central Highlands. He has been in Lima for twenty years, since he came from home He finished primary school there and he came to Lima for high school. He finished in the Colegio E_____ when he was around the age of 20. He finished the fifth year and entered the Coeducational School here.

He has been working here for seventeen years. He says: "It used to be obligatory to work here for one or two years as a nurse. Then you could go somewhere else. The salary is relatively low, the same for all nurses, 1500 soles a month. Yes, I have other work. It's at night in the Hospital del Empleado, from 7 to 7. They pay a little more than here: 1800 soles. I don't have any other work. I work there a week and I rest a week. The day shifts are six hours, and so the night nurse is compensated for his twelve-hour shift. My income is more or less enough when you put the two salaries together, but still it's a sacrifice. I'm married and we have three childrn of 9, 7, and 6."

Nurse Sara Delgado: She is 30 years old. She was born in a town on the South Coast. She has been in Lima for twenty-three years. She came for schooling. She had all of it here: "I haven't moved from Lima."

She graduated from high school at the age of 15. Then, she says, "I went to work as a nurse's aide in the Hospital Obrero. That was the way the nursing vocation grew inside me. You enter as an aide and you learn things little by little. You have to spend at least three months at it, and if you've learned how to do it they give you your appointment. When they appoint you as a nurse's aide it's a position and then they begin to pay you a little. They don't pay before that. If you don't learn, they dismiss you or they put you in housekeeping service. They observe you for three months. There's no examination but they appoint you on the basis of those observations.

"The nurse's aid job is the same as a nurse. I started on the two day shifts, from 7 to 1 and from 1 to 7. I worked for three years right there in the Hospital Obrero. I left that and began to study dress-making, but then I saw that I didn't like it. So I started in a retail store. I didn't like that either. I didn't feel comfortable. I'd gotten together the money I needed to buy my supplies and so I applied here.

"You have to buy uniforms. The Hospital gives them to us now, but in those days we had to buy everything. Now we have to buy shoes, stockings, underwear, and pajamas. We also have to buy our own watches and thermometers to replace the Hospital's if we break them.

"I will have been here eight years next April. They offer the job to all those of us who graduate high from the School. I began work immediately and I've worked here ever since.

"I make 1200 soles a month. Currently, I'm also working in the Hospital del Empleado at night. I work there as a private nurse to take care of one patient exclusively. It's called a "special nurse." I've also worked in the R_____ Clinic. It was just for short times, a month or a couple of weeks to take care of one patient. I'm also familiar with the D_____ Clinic. It's a clinic where they treat everything. I worked there as a special nurse. Also in the M_____ Clinic which is also a general clinic.

"The salary here is 1200 soles a month. I earn 1800 in the Hospital del Empleado, working there every two days. I'm married, with two children, 2 1/2 and 1 year and 2 months. My husband works in a commercial printer's. He earns 2000 a month. The combined income is enough. I have this job because I have to take care of my mother. She's not well. There are servants to take care of the children while I'm at work."

Nurse Miguel Esquivel: He is 51 years old. He was born in Qu_____, a town in the Central Highlands. He went to primary school there in Qu_____ where "fortunately I had a very good teacher." He came to Lima to go to high school He says, "I came because of the 1930 revolution. I was an orphan and the doors were closed to me. I got into this School a year after I finished high school.

"I went to work here after I graduated. There were sixteen of us, sixteen boys [sic] and eighteen or twenty women. Only four of the men stayed when they were asked by the Hospital management. I stayed because they asked me to.

"Here I earn 1258 soles a month with a bonus of 241. I don't work in other hospitals or clinics, but, yes, I work outside in my trade. I do a little business selling watches and jewelry. I work on commission. It's during my free shifts, about three or four hours. I earn about the same as here. Sometimes it's more and other times less. It's better than having a double shift. I don't have to run from one to another. I can rest and have a certain mental ease. I think that a nurse ought to be registered in one hospital and spend all his time there.

"I'm married with four children. A nurse is prevented from having his family. I didn't marry a nurse because I already knew all about it. My income has to take care of things. It isn't satisfying but it's enough. You can't compare it with the yankee style of life."

Nurse Rosa Frías: She is 28 years old. She was born in a town in the Central Highlands. She has been in Lima for eighteen years and had her primary and secondary schooling here.

She has been working here for eleven years. She says: "When I graduated from the School there were no vacancies here. I took care of a private patient in a home in San Isidro. I worked in that house with insulin therapy. Then Señorita Alicia called me here when there was a vacancy. I've worked here since then, but always with two jobs, the other in private homes and in clinics and always with mental patients. I've worked in the M_____ Clinic, the Military Hospital, the L_____ Clinic, the Hospital del Empleado, and a sanitarium for mental patients."

She earns 1250 soles monthly with a bonus of 241. Currently she is also working in the Hospital del Empleado on the other shift, with a free hour. She earns 2000. She says, "I make more in private homes, 300 for a night and 200 for a day. There are two nurses who work together and we divide it, with 100 for each one. At the Empleado the job and the salary are permanent. Private work is just from time to time.

"I'm married but I'm thinking about a divorce. I have a little boy of 3 1/2. My husband is in the lumber business. I don't know how much he makes, but it would be around 5000. His income is never fixed. Yes, our income is enough. It's very good. I take my whole salary to the bank, and I can pass it along to my relatives, my sister or anybody."

Nurse Amada Godoy: She is 27 years old. She was born in a city on the South Coast where she had her primary schooling. She has been in Lima for fourteen years. She came to attend high school.

She says: "Later a friend of mine told me about this School. She's still a nurse here. I came directly here. After I graduated, I was already used to the work. All fourteen of us who graduated togther stayed here to work, six are still here. The others are working in other hospitals."

She has been working here for six years and is earning 1250 soles a month with a bonus of 200. She does not have an outside job currently. She used to work in private homes, but not after she got married, because there was no time for it: "My husband is a TV technician. He's traveled a lot, to Venezuela and Colombia. He earns 3000. He also has another job, but that's separate. Our standard of living is comfortable. He always wants to improve it. I have two children, of 4 and 1. The income is comfortable, but not really. If you make more, you spend more."

Nurse Juan Hurtado: He is 28 years old. He was born in a city in the Central Highlands where he had both primary and secondary schooling. He has been in Lima for ten years. He came directly here [into the School] after he finished high school.

He has been working here for nine years. He is also working in the Hospital Seguro del Empleado. He makes 1500 here and 2000 at the Empleado, a little more with the bonus. He works there during the other shift, in the morning. He just works here in the afternoons. He is single, not engaged. His income is enough, then, because he lives here in the Hospital, on the second floor of Pavilion 6.

Nurse María Iglesias: She is 41 years old. She was born in a small city on the South Coast but had both primary and secondary education in Lima. She went to high school just to the second year. Then she went to a vocational school where she studied shorthand and typing. Then she came into the Nursing School here.

She has worked in several hospitals in Lima and Callao. She has been working here for just a year. She came to apply and since there was a vacancy the Director hired her. It was because she had been trained in this School. Besides, the work schedule is more comfortable than in other hospitals.

She earns 1475 a month. She has no other job outside, just work at home. She is married for the second time. She has two children, one from each marriage. The two are boys, one 14 years old and the other 4. Her salary isn't enough. If it were not for her husband's income, from his work as an employee, the month would end up with no money.

Nurse Teodora Justo: She is 32 years old. She was born in the capital of a Department in the Northern Highlands. She had three years of primary school at home, and finished it in Lima as she did with high school.

She has worked here fourteen years. She stayed on voluntarily after graduating from the School because she liked work in this

Hospital.

She is earning 1300 monthly. She also works in the Division of Surgery in the Hospital del Empleado where she earns 1900 soles. She also works in private clinics, but just for occasional day-work. She is married with a son of 7. The income is not enough. Her husband works, but she does not know how much he earns.

Nurse Héctor Lozada: He is 44 years old. He was born in Lima where he went to both primary and secondary school.

He has been working here for five years. He came when there was a vacancy and he petitioned the Director. Before that he has worked in the Hospital Dos de Mayo, in a mining company in the highlands, in public health for the Ministry of Health, also in the highlands, in the Miners' Bank, and in electric companies.

He works here in the afternoons and earns 1025 a month. From 9 to 12 he works in a collection company, in the division of municipal receipts with an income of 4000 soles a month. He is married and has three daughters of 17, 15, and 14. The income is modest. His wife works as a nurse with a monthly income of 3500.

Nurse Antonio Llona: He is 55 years old. He was born in the capital of a Department on the North Coast. He went to primary and secondary school in another northern city, and then he went to a commercial institute in Lima. He worked as a travel agent in the north before he entered the Nursing School here.

He has worked here continually from the time he graduated from the School, and he has also worked in a private clinic for some months. He earned 1050 soles monthly. He is married, with two daughters of 19 and 15. The income is not enough.

The nurses responded to the question, 6. "Why did you choose the occupation of nursing?" in the following terms:

Nurse Marta Arruga: Because it's a vocation. I always wanted to be a nurse from the time I was very small. Because it's a career that I look at as more appropriate for my sex as well as my character. From the time I was very small, I always liked helping my fellow humans and relieving pain.

Nurse Fernando Bustos: I have a cousin who is a doctor. He brought me to Lima to study for a year, to prepare myself to enter the Faculty of Dentistry. There was no time and so I studied the three years of nursing. Really, I didn't want to be a dentist. My cousin suggested it and I thought it would be a good profession.

The schedule was also convenient for me, and I didn't want to lose the habit of studying. I was thinking of preparing myself for a year in this School to enter [the University of] San Marcos. But there was no time for preparation between classes and practice. I kept putting it off till the next year. I thought it would be worth something, but it wasn't like that in anything. It wasn't worth anything to me, anything, anything. There's no future.

Nurse Santiago Cruz: To follow a career, to keep on studying, and to be able to work, because then I couldn't get into the Police School and I thought I'd take up something shorter like nursing. The idea came to me because I have a friend who was almost in the same class with me, and he advised me about the advantages and benefits. I thought it wasn't any use to dream about something else but that I should take up something more immediate.

Nurse Ricardo Chivas: Because, really, I liked it. My father worked here as a porter. It was a shorter course than anything else, and it was also easier.

Nurse Sara Delgado: I liked it. I had to work out of necessity. My family was poor, and after I got out of high school I had to work. I always wanted to be an *obstetriz* (licensed midwife), but there was no possibility of studying that. An obstetriz is the same thing as a *partera* (unlicensed midwife), but you have to take a university course. You get into La Maternidad de Lima [Lima Maternity Hospital], and you study there. There are 3 years of courses in the Faculty of Medicine of the University of San Marcos, and then one year of practice.

Nurse Miguel Esquivel: I fell into nursing. The universities closed down during the revolution [of 1930]. I wanted to go to the University. I liked science. Maybe I could have been a doctor. I was in Lima and there were a lot of young men looking for work, which was hard to find. I had two friends from home who were working here. I came to visit them. They were nurses. I came to Pavilion 6 with the spirit of an observer. It all caught my interest. I didn't have anything to do in Lima, and my friends invited me to stay for a couple of weeks. They gave me a bed there.

In those days, Dr. Valega [the Medical Director] was taking on attendants *ad honorem* [without pay]. I asked for work and the only thing I got was food. I spent a month like that. Dr. Caravedo was planning to open the School here at the time. All my friends avised me to matriculate here. I had been in the Nursing School at the Dos de Mayo for about three or four months the year before, and I knew about hospitals.

Nurse Rosa Frías: Because I'd always liked it from the time I was a girl. Well, it was my vocation not for economic reasons but because I liked it.

Nurse Amada Godoy: I liked it. I wanted to be an obstetriz, but first you have to be a nurse. When I graduated from here I couldn't keep on studying.

Nurse Juan Hurtado: It was by chance. I was preparing to go into Humanities at San Marcos. I didn't have time, and so I never applied. I came from my home town go to San Marcos, and then I met up with a friend from home who was working here. He told me about this School. He said it was a good one, and so I got interested in applying. That's the way I got into the School.

Nurse María Iglesias: Because from the time I was little I liked to help my school friends, especially if they needed first aid. I'd take them to a nearby drug store. I did the same thing at home. Besides having that hobby, I could make it a career without spending any money. I could do it in a short time, and that way I could crystalize my economic situation.

Nurse Teodora Justo: I liked to take care of patients.

Nurse Héctor Lozada: To serve my fellow humans and, especially, because I'd seen a case of this kind close to me.

Nurse Antonio Llona: I'd seen a friend killed in an auto accident. In that moment I wanted to be a doctor and I thought it was necessary for me to plan to study doctors and nurses.

To the question, 17, "How is the job of nurse here in general?", they responded as follows:

Nurse Marta Arruga: It's taking care of patients and doctors, administration, directing the attendants, seeing that the patients eat, seeing how they are, talking with them. It's also giving information about each patient to the doctors.

Sometimes you find it hard when they change you from one pavilion to another. Then you have to adjust to the patients, the doctors, and the activity of a new pavilion.

Nurse Fernando Bustos: It's almost that I don't see any advantage to it. The salary is bad. About the only advantage is the schedule.

Nurse Santiago Cruz: There's the head nurse, assistant nurse, and specialized nurses like those of us working here in insulin therapy. I don't want to be an assistant any more. The head has more years of service, more experience. You need to work five or six years to be a head. A head earns according to his years of service. He gets his percentage. I like that, more or less.

Nurse Ricardo Chivas: There are three categories: assistant, when you first start; pavilion nurse, which is what I am; and head of service, the most senior one. You're appointed head of service in a meeting of the nurses. It's according to the criterion of superiority.

Nurse Sara Delgado: A nurse has to do everything: she sees that food is given to the patients and she sees to administration. It's care and administration. There's one nurse for about 120 women patients. I'm in insulin therapy. I have ten patients in my care now, but we've had as many as fifteen. I'm here alone.

I prefer insulin therapy. I'm more independent here. I don't have to deal with the personnel. I can focus on taking care of my patients because it's a very delicate treatment.

Nurse Amada Godoy: It's what you've seen: first, taking care of patients in everything, and in relation to their treatment; and distributing clothing, medicine, and everything for the well being of the pavilion. Then we have to assist the doctor.

Generally there are two nurses but we have more here. We have to do everything, even to watch over labor therapy, and give each one work that she can do. And they can get violent, so we have to see that there are no disturbances. There's a radio, too, and you have to play soft music. You've got to look after the cleaning, too: the windows and the doors. And you have to call the carpenter if something needs to be repaired. Also clothing: you have to see that it's delivered and that the patients change their clothes.

Nurse Juan Hurtado: I want to obey everything that's ordered by the bosses, the doctors. Yes, I like it. Habit turns into liking.

Nurse María Iglesias: It's good, but you have to do everything.

Nurse Teodora Justo: It's all right.

Nurse Héctor Lozada: It depends on the number of patients. For example, this pavilion has 80 patients.

Nurse Antonio Llona: There's a lot of activity.

In response to the question of *how is the job?*, I expected possible statements like, for example, "it's interesting," "there's little remuneration," "it has a lot of responsibility," "it's satisfying," "it's not what I wanted to do," and so on. Consequently, I was surprised that many (but, of course, not all) of the subjects chose to specify their duties or to give lists of the stages of the nursing career. It is possible that there exists more anxiety beneath the surfaces of the responses, that is, as indicated by the silences, than in the words themselves. So it is that many subjects unconsciously hear another question, and respond to *what?* instead of *how?*. Also, as it will be seen in what is to come, some of the nurses appear to search for security precisely in the tasks which have almost nothing to do with patient care, like administrative duties. Contradictions can exist among the different tasks. An enumeration of such tasks assists the avoidance of evaluating them. In this respect Menzies Lyth (1988:51) says:

> The core of the anxiety situation for the nurse lies in her relation with the patient. The closer and more concentrated this relationship, the more the nurse is likely to experience the impact of anxiety. The nursing service attempts to protect her from the anxiety by splitting up her contact with patients. It is hardly too much to say that the nurse does not nurse patients. The total workload of a ward or department is broken down into lists of tasks, each of which is allocated to a particular nurse. She performs her patient-centered tasks for a large number of patients--perhaps as many as all the patients in the ward, often thirty or more. As a corollary, she performs only a few tasks for, and has restricted contact with, any one patient. This prevents her from coming effectively into contact with the totality of any one patient and his illness and offers some protection from the anxiety this arouses.

The subjects expressed their feelings about their profession better in their responses to the questions, 22, "What qualifications should a person have to be a nurse?" and 23, "What qualifications should a person have to work as a nurse here?":

Nurse Marta Arruga: The essential thing is for her to have the vocation. Then she should have certain personal characteristics like a good character, being generous, disinterested.

The first thing should-- It's that some are afraid. They have to get used to the kinds of patients here. There are all kinds. She has to have a special character. Some patients require patience. She has to have a lot of patience. Some are like babies, some are violent. You can't control them without teaching them to respect the professional person, the nurse. And above all it's necessary for a person to like this work with these patients.

Nurse Fernando Bustos: They tell you when you get in that you have to have the vocation. But you can work hard in any profession that you enter. It doesn't make any difference. Any person can do it.

Just the desire to work and be responsible. If you're a nurse you could get in here. Some are afraid, but when they get used to it they're not any more. You have to have patience. Anybody can adapt.

Nurse Santiago Cruz: First, a spirit of observation, being an observer. Next, punctuality. You have to be worthy of confidence. You need to be handy. Method.

Everyone thinks he can adapt to any circumstance. You come in as a student and you get to adapt yourself. A person can get used to any situation. You adapt for three years, and if you don't during this time you leave. Or you finish up and then go to work in other hospitals. It depends on whether or not you like the Hospital or being with mental patients.

Nurse Ricardo Chivas: You always have to know how to understand the patient. Some are temperamental, others are passive or active. You have to know how to deal with them and lead them. The nurse needs understanding for the patient. You have to understand what a patient is, that he can give you a slap or a kick. They hurt a lot of nurses. You have to understand how this comes from the illness. Psychopaths are lucid but they have another way of behaving.

Nurse Sara Delgado: A vocation, her health, and her responsibility.

Vocation is the willingness that you have to give attentive care.

You have to have good nerves, a well formed personality, because things here influence you a lot. You have to be a person who is adaptable to the kind of place it is.

Nurse Miguel Esquivel: First, vocation, a spirit of sacrifice, but not too much.

It's important to have character, tact for dealing with patients. You need characteristics that are helpful in keeping up a pavilion. We're like householders. We have to do everything. It's a heavy responsibility. It's not easy if a person is not in condition to do it.

Nurse Rosa Frías: She has to have a lot of vocation, patience, a good character for taking care of patients. A bad tempered person can't take care of patients.

You have to be specialized. A lot of people want to be nurses, but not mental nurses. You have to study in this School. Any person who graduates can work as a mental nurse. You leave it early if you don't like it. They give the worst jobs to students, bathing incontinent patients, and things like that.

Nurse Amada Godoy: Above all, vocation, a spirit of understanding, and inspiring confidence in the patient, because otherwise you're lost for him.

Just any person couldn't work here. Nurses from other hospitals can't. They're afraid of the patients. They look at them timidly and think that somebody's going to hurt them. If you study in this School you can adapt. But the others don't know the patients. Women who have just worked in women's pavilions are afraid of working in men's pavilions. A girl went to Pavilion 6 and a boy who always behaved himself took advantage of her, because she didn't know the service, and he hit her. They know when you're afraid and they get aggressive. This happens to students from the other schools. Once a patient hit a student, and when the nurse asked her why, the patient said: "It's because she's afraid of me, and so I made her more afraid."

Nurse Juan Hurtado: He has to have character, a special personality, patience above all. A temperament that's capable of suffering. Those are the basic qualifications, especially for psychiatric nursing.

Nurse María Iglesias: Abnegation, understanding, and being

charitable.

She should have more patience and understanding of the patients themselves, and be with them in the sense of their illness itself.

Nurse Teodora Justo: To have aptitude for giving care to these kinds of patients.

Not to have prejudices or fears.

Nurse Héctor Lozada: A physique, culture, vocation, and education.

Size and having knowledge of psychology.

Nurse Llona: Abnegation, sacrifice. Not thinking like the "Rotary." You give your all to the Hospital and from it you don't even receive an honorable compensation.

Culture, understanding for the mental patient because he's a human being.

In these materials a certain emphasis on "vocation" as a qualification for professional success is to be noted. The frequent repetition of this response, and the almost mechanical manner with which it is delivered, suggest that it is a bit of ideology which is taught in the School and learned, without great reflection, in order to satisfy the instructional staff. Menzies Lyth (1988:61-62) sees such idealization and undervaluation of the possibilities of personal development as a defense against tension, as in the use of phrases like "nurses are born, not made" or "nursing is a vocation." She points out:

> This amounts to a kind of idealization of the potential nursing recruit, and implies a belief that responsibility and personal maturity cannot be "taught" or even greatly developed. As a corollary, the training system is mainly orientated to the communication of essential facts and techniques, and pays minimal attention to teaching events orientated to personal maturation within the professional setting.

In the context of the qualifications that the nurses had in mind, let us now examine their responses to the questions, 24, "What are the nurse's tasks?" and 25, "Which do you like more? Which less?":

Nurse Marta Arruga: First, in the morning you receive personnel and distribute the work. You receive the watchman's report. Then you have to make your rounds all around the pavilion to see if there's something new. Next you get things ready for the doctor, the forms. If it's electroshock day, you need to get ready for them. If there's analysis, you have to see that they don't eat breakfast. You have to give out medications, and then you make rounds with the doctors. You make out prescriptions for the doctors to sign. Then come the injections. But before that you have to see to the attendants' work and the patients' condition. Then you do the treatment forms for each patient. And then comes lunch time. Sometimes it's necessary to feed negative patients. You also have to instruct the attendants. There are many other things: sending food out, asking for keys, soap, and clothes. That's not all.

I like injections the most, and making rounds with the doctors because you learn more when you're with them, electroshock treatments, passing out pills and vitamins--because if these things aren't given to them they don't get better.

I don't like asking the administration for things. And also when a patient is moribund, because although you see it all the time you don't want it.

Nurse Fernando Bustos: I arrive and give insulin at 6:30. Then I have breakfast and come back. We have a nurses' dining room across from the kitchen. I think our food is sixth category, very bad and heavy. It's a skimpy breakfast: a small cup of milk and two small pieces of bread just with butter. It's a little better than breakfast for the patients. They bring you better food for lunch. Well, I come back to the insulin room and I have to control the patients until they enter coma. I control the coma, and if it's bad I cut it in less than an hour. If it's going well I don't interrupt it for an hour. It's not good to hold it more than an hour, except in special cases. Then we see to it that the patient eats well. After that the work is over. I have to prepare treatment lists. There's a form for each patient. That's all. I like controlling the coma, and sometimes trying out certain methods according to what the book says.

I dislike almost none of them in insulin therapy. Well, I don't like pavilion service. Señor Muelle is the head, because of his seniority. Before he came, there wasn't a head nurse. Only some of them have this title. It's been a while since I've done that kind of work. I like to make cures. We don't like to work in the afternoon because there's nothing to do and we get bored.

Nurse Santiago Cruz: The job is working in the insulin therapy room, giving care to patients in insulin therapy while that treatment goes on, and later too. You have to watch and control the comas, see that they eat, and leave reports for the afternoon nurse if it's especially necessary to watch certain patients. You have to be very careful with the patients here. We also help if they need us somewhere else.

I like everything the same, because it's all necessary.

Our work is different from that of the attendants. Cleaning lavatories is disgusting and some don't like it. Some are afraid and that's because they prefer one type of work over another. The nurse's duties include not just giving care to patients but guiding the attendants. In medicine or surgery there are things that a person likes better. Here it's all the same. Not every nurse can give anesthesia or handle the instruments. There's more specialization and more experience in these other fields than here.

Nurse Ricardo Chivas: Giving care to the patient, administration of the service. You have to see to the needs of the service as a whole. He's like the father at home who sees if a patient needs clothing, what his condition is. You have to look for certain things and ask the administration for them. We have an insulin room with one nurse. He's Señor Orellana and comes only in the morning. We have four patients in insulin therapy.

I like the technical part most. I've been working for three years in insulin therapy in Pavilions 12, 2, and 18. When you move into the head's job, then you have to be busy with administrative duties.

Nurse Sara Delgado: First I come and see if a patient's in good health, with no fever or cold. Then insulin treatment is applied. After that you tell the patients to return to their beds. You have to take care of their personal cleanliness. They put their pajamas on and go to bed. Then you observe the precoma. All the symptoms have to be recorded until it's seen that they're entering the coma. Then you control it according to time, because a patient has to remain in that state for an hour. It's interrupted with glucose. It's given in the form of syrup. You take them to the bathroom and give them showers, and then they come back for a hot drink. You have to dress them and get them ready to go to lunch in the dining room, and see that they eat everything. Then you give them something to entertain them. If no other symptom appears, you give them to the afternoon nurse. If some patient is disturbed, you need to report this to her so she can note it down and take care. After that, the job is over. You have to prepare forms on coma days, how many comas, the quality of the glucose, the syrup, the insulin.

I like it all, the whole process. Nobody shows the same symptoms.

They vary, just like the reactions vary.

Nurse Miguel Esquivel: Doing everything, in the office, the nurses' station, in the therapy rooms.

Everything's obligatory. I like injections and records. I've worked on statistics now and then. I like to fill out forms, take care of the office. Which less? I can't think of anything.

Nurse Rosa Frías: I like to assist the doctors. I don't like to take charge of the attendants. In other hospitals nurses don't have to see to the cleaning.

I like to be with the doctors so I can get more knowledge, and I like to give treatments to the patients. I like everything that has to do with patients. I don't like bothering about the cleaning.

Nurse Amada Godoy: I like treatment for the patients, and also medical consultation. You watch behavior and you evaluate the patient. You have to provide information so that the doctors know how to vary medication. You also watch when a patient is given leave or is discharged. The treatment isn't just giving pills. Students give out pills but they don't watch the effects in the patients. You have to open your eyes to see the reactions. Everything's related. There's nothing that disgusts me, that I dislike.

In some pavilions they don't fill out forms, but that's where there aren't any medications and they don't give treatment. But where I've worked we've had to control treatment strictly. In Pavilion 8, on outpatient days, we've taken care of forty-five or fifty patients in electroshock. This pavilion [the one in which the interview is taking place] has more outpatients. In Pavilion 1 they also have them, but not as many. Here today we've had ten patients. Dr. Urteaga likes to take care of a large number of people. It only takes two minutes for each one. Everything's arranged to save time. The attendants are trained for the work. There are two rooms, one for males and the other for women.

Nurse Juan Hurtado: In the first place, to watch the patient's health. Here the work is limited to giving patient care in whatever can happen immediately. They almost don't get treatment, given their number and the deteriorated state of many of them.

I've always liked work in insulin therapy, because I've done it since I was a student and I've almost come to specialize in it. I've given almost half of my time to it over the last four or five years. I do it in the Seguro del Empleado.

Nurse María Iglesias: She should be conscientious, punctual. She should carry out all the doctor's orders.
I like all the duties. They're all agreeable. I don't dislike any.

Nurse Teodora Justo: Carrying out obligations.
They're all the same.

Nurse Héctor Lozada: Carrying out professional orders, taking care of patients, having respect for superiors.
I like being in direct contact with patients. I don't like office duties.

Nurse Antonio Llona: Conscientiousness, sacrifice, abnegation, in all, everything that one can give of oneself.
I like being conscientious and giving care. I like everything. [He smiles.]

To the question, 36, "What is the best aspect of the job? The worst? What advantages does it have?", which was only posed to some of the subjects, they responded:

Nurse Marta Arruga: That they give us a bed, a room, and that we don't have many expenses. It would be economic. The worst is that we don't have protection when a patient attacks. A patient took off a male nurse's ear. They can kill a nurse. A patient threw a stone at a female nurse's back and she came down with tuberculosis.[6]

Nurse Fernando Bustos: The satisfaction of seeing that a patient has recuperated. In insulin therapy we see the partial or total reestablishment of a patient who comes in quite agitated. The worst is for men. We always resent it because sometimes the group of doctors, the ones who direct nurses, show a distinct preference for the feminine sex. Almost nobody wants to get the nurse's certificate because it's exclusively for a woman. It says "*interesada*" ["concerned," with a feminine gender suffix; the masculine gender form would be "*interesado*"] on it, and no man wants to have that. When they ask for nurses in the provinces, they ask for women.

Nurse Santiago Cruz: I can't answer. There almost isn't any advantage. They're all disadvantages. Maybe the schedule? There are so many disadvantages. For example, the work is very demanding in the sense of being present, because there's the greatest pressure to be here because it's necessary. The remuneration, also, because a nurse has a disturbing job. We also need convenient ways to come and go from work. In the event a person is single, if he has no family, who's he going to spend some time with for relaxation, for mental hygiene?

Nurse Ricardo Chivas: They teach you to know something about health, and this is useful at home if something happens. It's beneficial to know something about this specialty outside, or at home, if somebody has trouble. The worst aspect is the economic part. It's not in agreement with what it should be.

Nurse Sara Delgado: The nurse is in charge. She's the topmost person in the service. She earns the most. She has the respect and obedience of all the attendants and the patients. The disadvantage is that almost all the responsibility for the service is in the nurse's hands.

What were the nurses' plans for the future? We turn now to the responses to the questions, 14, "How long do you expect to continue work here?", 15, "Do you want to continue your occupation your whole life? If not, what do you want to do?", and 16, "Do you want to continue in psychiatric nursing?":

Nurse Marta Arruga: While I--if God gives me the strength, all my life if I can.

Yes, in nursing.

Yes.

Nurse Fernando Bustos: I'm going to work six years more. I can't finish earlier. Later on I'll have to be in class all day [studying engineering], and then I'll be working here at night, if they let me. If not, I'll be an attendant. They earn half the salary but it makes no difference.

No.

No.

Nurse Santiago Cruz: If I found better work I'd leave, because I don't plan to stay here forever. I could get out if I were to find something. I'd like to improve the situation.

By all means I plan to work till I can find another career. If I don't find something, I'll stay. I'd like to get into the veterinary faculty in San Marcos. It's a five-year course, but it's an occupation out in the open air. I'm getting ready and studying so I won't forget things. I'd like to get in next year. I plan to continue working while I'm studying. I'll have to arrange a night schedule, or if I don't get that I'll look for a job in some other hospital or in public assistance. When there's a vacancy they'll let me know.

Yes, if I don't get what I hope. Our specialty is psychiatry, although we can work in other specialties too.

Nurse Ricardo Chivas: Until I stop with my thirty years.

Just at retirement age. After that I'll do whatever comes along. I'd look for something that would help.

Yes.

Nurse Sara Delgado: I'll be working just this year. After that, I'll just stay on in the Empleado as a night guard. I won't work in the daytime. They want to prevent us from working in two places, but how can you live with just one job? I'll have to leave because of that.

Yes.

No, I now prefer general nursing. I'll work any place, but not in a psychiatric service. It's very sad to be taking care of these cases and to see that so many of them stay for so many months recuperating, and that others never get well.

Nurse Miguel Esquivel: I'm going to complete the required time of thirty years. Then I'm going to work outside in my trade [the sale of watches and jewelry], but I'll enlarge the business. I could stay here, but why? If they paid me double it would be good, but otherwise why stay?

Nurse Rosa Frías: Always. I don't plan to leave because I like this Hospital a lot. Although you learn more in other places, I'd rather stay here because I like it. There isn't another like it.

Nurse Amada Godoy: Just for this year. My husband doesn't want me to work. I'd be at home.

I'd like to stay here, but circumstances oblige me. The two babies need their mother.

Yes.

Nurse Juan Hurtado: I still haven't decided on the time.

It depends on whether or not I see a better occupation. I could get out.

Yes, as long as I keep on as a nurse. I'd like to study another career outside nursing. I don't have plans right now. My double occupation [shifts at two hospitals] doesn't allow me to do anything this year. I'm planning to leave one of the jobs. I have to see which will give me more time for studying. I want to study in the humanities, especially philosophy applied to education.

Nurse Héctor Lozada: Three years.

Yes, I have a plan to carry out in the three years. Without leaving my profession I plan to take up agricultural activities.

Yes.

All the subjects had had a wide variety of experiences in the different pavilions of the Hospital and, of course they had their preferences and antipathies. I asked them, 18, "In which pavilions have you worked?" and 19, "Which do you prefer and why?" They responded:

Nurse Marta Arruga: In all of them. When we would go on night guard duty, we had to go around to all of the pavilions. We even went to 4 [the large pavilion of male charity patients]. That was the way it used to be. We stopped that five years ago. Now we divide it between the men and the women. There are just two who do this work alone.

The work is the same in all pavilions. I like this one because I work here now. I don't like Pavilion 10 [the male pavilion for patients with tuberculosis; 11 is the female counterpart] because it doesn't have facilities. There's no clothing. I'm not afraid of the disease, tuberculosis, because a person can catch it everywhere. In 5 [the large pavilion for female charity patients] you can't say that it's hard to adapt, even though it's like 4, because the women patients try to help you.

Nurse Fernando Bustos: I've worked in all of them. That is, I've been in all the men's pavilions except 10. I haven't worked in 14 [for children], because male nurses don't work there.

I'm staying here because of the work in insulin therapy. This work is the best in the Hospital. I like this pavilion [where the interview is taking place] because of the medical personnel. They're more understanding, younger, and they're better at letting you alone, especially Dr. Bueno whom I've known for years. It's very good and he's been here for three years. Here they leave you free. You can read books and apply what you've read. Dr. Vega in Pavilion [n] is very strict and doesn't let you. Pavilion 4 is forgotten by the whole Hospital.

They're the same to me. I don't like Pavilion [n], or the service, or those I worked with. I don't like anything there. The nursing personnel are ancient. I've worked in 4, but I wouldn't like to go back there because I couldn't work in insulin therapy. I'd go anywhere there was insulin therapy. In [n] there's a doctor who doesn't treat the nurses well. Everybody is complaining. I'd prefer not to work there at all.

Nurse Santiago Cruz: I've worked in all the men's pavilions.

I prefer it here because here there's more work and you keep busy. There's more treatment in comparison with the others. The others are boring. Here there's more movement. It's more lively, cleaner. There's more space. The rest of the pavilions are all the same. I've worked a lot in 4 and they've never attacked me.

Nurse Ricardo Chivas: In all the men's pavilions. I've been working here for a month.

It's about the same, the same kind of work, the same specialty. They're all the same. A nurse is indifferent if there isn't something personal between him and the doctor. 10 is all right because the same disease can be found everywhere. In 4 it often depends on how you deal with the patients.

Nurse Sara Delgado: In all of them. Once the administration wanted to send me to 4 with a male nurse but I protested. It's a terrible place, but maybe there wouldn't have been any problem because it seems like male patients obey women more than men.

I prefer 12 and 18. 12 [a men's pavilion, with its counterpart, 13, for women] is an admissions pavilion and you can see cases from the beginning. You see how a patient comes in and how he recuperates. It's the most interesting in all aspects. You learn more. 18 has all the conveniences. It's a service for paying patients and insurance cases. It has its treatments.

I dislike none of them. In 10 and 11 you really don't run any risks. That disease exists in all the pavilions. It's silly because it's just in the name, in the fact that those pavilions are reserved for patients with tuberculosis. I don't like working there because there's no water. There isn't any equipment to get the work done. It doesn't have clothes. The Charity Society is so poor it can't give us DDT, cleaning fluid, and so on, to clean up those places. Who's going to like working there? 4 and 5 are the pavilions that are in the worst condition. The others don't have all the conveniences, except for one thing or another that save the situation.

Nurse Miguel Esquivel: I've worked almost everywhere. I just haven't worked in the kitchen, the laboratory, the drug dispensary, and the chapel. I've worked everywhere else, of course in the men's part.

I'm a combat soldier. I have no preference. I don't say that this pavilion is dirty and that I don't like it. The charity regimen is better because, with paying patients, the patients' relatives bother you and you can't attend to your duties. I like it better here. I like to be useful where I'm needed most. The need is greatest here.

Nurse Rosa Frías: In all of them.

It's the same. They're all mental patients and you give them the same care. I don't like Pavilion [n] because of the doctor. I had a disagreement with him. Other pavilions have more work. This pavilion has more activity. As for the rest, it's routine.

Nurse Amada Godoy: I've worked in 1, 6, and 8.

They're the same. Not really, but as far as the work goes. The work's the same.

There aren't many conveniences in the charity regimen. This pavilion is better because the patients pay. There you have to fight to get something. Here, when something runs out it's easier to get it again. Those problems don't come up here because the patients pay for their medications.

Some pavilions are completely bad, like 11. It's for both charity and paying patients but it's contagious and it doesn't have any conveniences. It's completely deteriorated. 4 isn't a pavilion but an asylum. There's no clothing, food, and personnel. 5 is like 4 [which contained 233 patients], because it lacks almost everything and there are 192 women patients and one nurse. Even food is scarce. There are 192 women and, what's worse, they fight. They fight and break each other's heads, and with so few personnel nothing can be done. They are deteriorated people, deformed, because they're abandoned. They're chronic and incurable. They've had all the treatments and haven't responded.

Nurse Juan Hurtado: In all except for the women's.

There's almost no preference. They're all the same. Sometimes, from the point of view of an administrator, there are problems. For example, you'd have interest in this pavilion if it weren't that there are no materials to do the work or conveniences to do something for the patients. I prefer 18 from the administrative point of view because it's better. There's better discipline. It begins with the doctors. They're interested in the patients. That's the best way.

It isn't that I like 4 less, but you have trouble there because you can't carry on with high spirits. There's no clothing, food, water, and a whole lot of things.

While the nurses can localize their preferences, perhaps only to comply with the task given by the question, at the same time there exists in many of the responses the sense of "it's all the same to me." This can represent detachment and the denial of emotions, as indicated by Menzies Lyth (1988:53):

> A necessary psychological task for the entrant into any profession that works with people is the development of adequate professional detachment. He must learn, for example, to control his feelings, refrain from excessive involvement, avoid disturbing identifications, maintain his professional independence against manipulation and demands for unprofessional behaviour. To some extent the reduction of individual distinctiveness aids detachment by minimizing the mutual interaction of personalities, which might lead to "attachment". It is reinforced by an implicit operational policy of "detachment". "A good nurse doesn't mind moving." A "good nurse" is willing and able without disturbance to move from ward to ward or even hospital to hospital at a moment's notice. . . . The pain and distress of breaking relationships and the importance of stable and continuing relationships are implicitly denied by the system, although they are often stressed personally--that is, nonprofessionally--by people in the system.

The nurses also had their preferences regarding the patients with whom they liked working, accompanied of course by the same detachment, as can be seen in their responses to the questions, 43, "What type of patient do you like most, and why?" and 44, "What type of patient do you like least, and why?":

Nurse Marta Arruga: Those who behave themselves and cooperate in their treatment, but aren't submissive. You can do something for them. In chronic cases, you can help but not much.

There are patients who know what they're doing but are rude and insolent. G_____ wants everything when he asks for it. Some are imperious and abuse the attendants. G_____ is lucid but demanding. He could help but he doesn't. He's the only one.

Nurse Fernando Bustos: The type of illness? I like to deal with patients who have neurosis, the ones with small problems that can be treated with psychotherapy, because the ones with schizophrenia--well! I like the boys here. I like them more because they are the patients who have a lot of hope in a cure. In general they have acute psychosis. They're treatable. With chronic patients, well, you can't do very much.

I don't like the epileptics. They have a sticky personality. They like to bother you. There are no strong epileptics here, but we have D_____. [I ask about R_____.] Of course, R_____ certainly has the personality but I've never seen him in a crisis.

Nurse Santiago Cruz: None of them are the same. Who's not going to like working with patients who cooperate, ones who aren't disturbed? But I have to work with all of them, and they're all the same to me. I don't care whether they're clean or messy, disturbed or calm, their social class, the social scale, whether or not they're white, because in this Hospital there are all kinds. We can't think about differences.

Personally, there aren't any that I don't like.

Nurse Ricardo Chivas: It's not important to us. In every pavilion there are all types, and we have to be with them all and give them care. You get used to dealing with all of them. I'm indifferent. I like to help patients to raise their spirits, reestablish themselves. That's my goal. You have to deal with them and help in any way you can.

The disturbed ones are the most uncomfortable and dangerous. But you have to resolve that and treat them all the same.

Nurse Sara Delgado: I like attending in medicine, surgery, and with cases of trauma. I very much like taking care of patients with disturbances of conduct, psychopaths, as they say, because I think that in this role the nurse can help in the patient's improvement. She can lend her services and they aren't difficult to treat.

I don't like the catatonics because they are incontinent with urine and feces.

Nurse Miguel Esquivel: I don't know any patient that I could say I like. I have to take care of all of them and I do it.

The alcoholics are undesirable for me. I have the obligation of taking care of all of them, but it's easier for me to say which I don't like.

Nurse Rosa Frías: I like the paranoid type of schizophrenic because it's easier to give them treatment. You can see the improvement.

I don't like the psychopaths. They seem to me like the worst because they like to hurt. They're always hitting and insulting the other patients. And they are conscious of what they're doing.

Nurse Amada Godoy: Almost all of them are mentally retarded. They are harmless. I like the lucid ones more, because the retarded patients can't converse with you, although they're tame. Some of them are totally oriented and only get bad occasionally.

Some feel persecuted and those are the ones who can hurt you. It's a matter of getting used to it. The psychopaths and the epileptics are the worst. They start insulting you from the time they come into the Hospital. They bother you, but not so much that you have an aversion for them.

Nurse Juan Hurtado: I'd rather take care of a mental patient. I like acute cases of schizophrenia in which you see the best prognosis. They recuperate more easily.

I don't like the mentally retarded because you can't get changes in their behavior or in what is called mental recuperation.

Now that we have an idea of what the nurses had to say about their tasks and preferences, we come to the matter of how they evaluate their preparation for their work. A sense of this can be drawn from their responses to the questions, 26, "Have you received any special training to carry out the work of a psychiatric nurse?" and 27, "Are you satisfied with the training? If not, what would you have liked?

Nurse Marta Arruga: Just the courses they give everybody here. Specialization occurs with the time in service you have here and with practice.

With the courses? Yes, some of them, but in others the instructors are not competent. We all take the same courses. Professional formation takes place in hospitals, each one according to his or her specialty. Some get more interested in psychiatry. We do our practice while we're taking the course. I think there ought to be special courses to develop personnel to give treatment according to the character of the patients. They ought to teach the care you have to give them, how to act with them, as a specialized course. They ought to teach symptoms to distinguish one diagnosis from another, and how to make observations on each patient. They also ought to teach this to general nurses because these things can appear in a general hospital. It's good to have general nurses passing through here so they won't maltreat patients later. They're afraid and they have strange ideas, so when they come here they learn that it's something else.

Nurse Fernando Bustos: Yes, they give it to us. The course on psychiatry is more intense. We take a course that's called "Art of Nursing" that deals with what a nurse has to do. Each school has it, but they give it to us with application to mental patients. The nurses also train us in practice. You learn more in pavilions than in school. It happens to us like that for the whole three years, for about six hours every day. The School produces nurses who are more specialized, though they finish with the title, "General Nurse."

I think that the training isn't enough. Some courses are good and others miss the mark. You have to learn from experience. Some courses in medicine taught by doctors are very good, but others are weaker. The courses could improve. There's too much disinterest in the School.

Nurse Santiago Cruz: Yes, here in the School they give us care of mental patients. They give us classes on admission, diagnosis, the precautions you need to take with the patient and his relatives. It's a long chapter in the text they give us. I don't remember the author's name. The title is "Care of Mental Patients" ["Atención de los enfermos mentales"]. It's one section of the course. They give us pediatrics, obstetrics, and mental patients. The first year is the care and treatment of patients; the second is medicine and surgery; and the third is practice.

Yes, I'm satisfied.

Nurse Ricardo Chivas: Just in this School a part of the course has to do with psychiatric nursing. You specialize here. For emergencies you also need to know the other branches. We have special courses, but we can specialize in other brances. A lot of nurses go to work in other hospitals.

The training here is very solid. There's much material to work on.

Nurse Sara Delgado: Yes, we take a course in psychology. It's deeper than the other courses they give other nurses. And the doctors give us classes on the services and prepare us in a way that the others don't get. They give talks to us and short courses.

Yes, I'm satisfied with general nursing. If they made us into

> specialists there wouldn't be room for everyone. We could only work in this Hospital. Almost all the nurses in the Military Hospital, in almost all the services, are graduates from here. There are many of us in the Empleado. These are new hospitals and when they opened many graduates from here applied for jobs and got them.
>
> Nurse Miguel Esquivel: This School was the first for specialists. We received a general training. Now they're careless about the specialty. I think that the training ought to be general, but they should have a special course and, of course, good practice. It has to be more intensive, but this can be given in the kind of practice that you get here.
>
> No. It's missing something because the students need more practice and less laziness. There's a course on the art of nursing where they've doubled the part that deals with the history of nursing.
>
> Nurse Amada Godoy: Here in the School the course is special-general, but there's a short course. And you learn during practice because you always go to the pavilions. There's a little fear at the beginning, but you get used to it. These patients need more care and vigilance. You have to give them more attention than other patients. Nurses get to love them.
>
> Nurse Juan Hurtado: We could say that we're specialized from having done our studies in a psychiatric hospital. I liked surgery. When I was in training there was no operation that I didn't see.
>
> The training is good, more or less. They give formal courses, and they give practice in the pavilions. The program is general but we learn more about this specialty because we live here. If a student is interested, he gets it because he lives here.

Thus, nurses received much more psychiatric and psychological training in the Hospital's School than nurses in other schools; however, it seems that some of them have strong wishes to go deeper in this direction. They depart from the pattern, described by Kalkman (1974:224), of the traditional relations between doctor and nurse:

> The psychiatric nurse first became involved in the treatment of mentally ill patients because, other than the psychiatrist, the nurse was the only health professional directly concerned with patient care who had a knowledge of drugs, their uses, and their desirable and undesirable effects. This attribute took precedence over any knowledge of psychology or psychiatry that a nurse might have. In

> the late nineteenth and early twentieth century the extent of this knowledge was very little or none. The traditional doctor-nurse relationship obtained in this period, in which the physician diagnosed and prescribed the drug and the nurse administered the drug to the patient and reported its effects to the physician.

The nurses, like the attendants, remembered their first experiences in the Hospital and spoke about their fears in their responses to the questions, 53, "What happened to you when you came to the Hospital to work the first time?," 54, "What things do you think are most important for getting used to it?," and 55, "What were your greatest difficulties?":

> Nurse Marta Arruga: Well, a certain--a little nervous because I wasn't familiar with it. It was the first time I saw a mental hospital and I had a certain fear. But after two days, then I was walking all around the Hospital with no fear.
>
> That the fears go away and a person gets to know everything. I got used to it and lost my fear by getting to know the Hospital.

> Nurse Fernando Bustos: I wasn't afraid, or anything, because I had friends. They oriented me. And they prepared me for the kind of patient that I was going to deal with, so that I developed overconfidence. When I was attacked by one of them I had to change.
>
> You need a good education in the Nursing School. But the older nurses are more important than anyone else that teaches you.
>
> I only had a problem in the second year with one instructor. She bothered the boys a lot. She was interested in asylum politics and our veneration.

> Nurse Santiago Cruz: When I was a student, it seemed to me like an inexplicable thing when I realized that so many patients were so different from what I saw on the streets outside the Hospital. So I felt sad to find them restrained and isolated in a morally deplorable position and situation.
>
> Adaptation and the presentations the instructors gave us, and staying with everybody else as nurses. In a group you feel better, more secure. But alone, imagine!
>
> It was in service, in the pavilions where I was there were very disturbed patients.

> Nurse Ricardo Chivas: At the beginning it always affects you.

You suffer the consequences of the work a little, the School's discipline. It's a bit uncomfortable. At the beginning you're afraid. Outside they always ask you, "How are the crazy people?" They think that everybody is tied up. But you get used to it.

For example, always dealing with the rest of your superiors. You get yourself going around confidently.

The difficulty is being interned in the School. Students could go out only once a week. Now it's changed a little.

Nurse Sara Delgado: I was timid, nervous, restrained. It lasted a month and then I adapted. I wasn't afraid any more, either of the personnel or the patients. When you have that, you've won everything here.

It was that I missed my parents, because I'd never been apart from them before.

Nurse Miguel Esquivel: I felt I didn't like it. It was natural because I wasn't used to it. Little by little you adapt to the situation. Now I've been here for thirty years.

Controlling your own will is important.

Nurse Rosa Frías: I was sad because I came alone and nobody from my family came with me. I applied by myself. All my friends came with their relatives.

I got used to it fast. I didn't go outside. I stayed in the Hospital. I'm friendly and I got used to it fast. It was easy.

Nurse Amada Godoy: We came to the School. It had a pleasant atmosphere, protecting. The students were good, friendly. We went to class and we got used to it. After four months we went to the services. It wasn't a shock because we'd got used to it. In Pavilion 7 they were peaceful because it's a pavilion with physical illnesses. The transition wasn't sudden and we could adapt.

The important thing is adaptation, the spirit of understanding.

There was no difficulty.

Nurse Juan Hurtado: A person always feels strange when he comes in. It's a shock. You find yourself surrounded by ones who are known outside as crazy people. When you find yourself with the patients you feel strange, that they are abnormal.

Nurse María Iglesias: I felt afraid. I noticed every movement and the patients' ideas.

You need strength of will and resignation to adapt.

Nurse Teodora Justo: I felt timid.
You become familiar with the Hospital atmosphere little by little.
It cost me tears because of the treatment I received from the advanced students.

Nurse Héctor Lozada: The patients thought I was a patient because I didn't dress in white.
I felt ill at ease and with a certain fear of patients.
Nurses in those days had little psychiatric knowledge.

Nurse Antonio Llona: I had a certain fear. I thought the patients could be like drunks who aren't aware of their actions.
What is important is your friends and dealing with your superiors.
I had no difficulty. I got used to it fast.

As in the interviews with other population categories, the last question put to the nurses was, 56, "Suppose that I were a new nurse who had just come into the job, what advice would you give me for getting used to it more rapidly?" They answered as follows:

Nurse Marta Arruga: You have to know the service. I'd tell you the characteristics of the patients, and not to be afraid of them. To make frienships so as to have a pleasant life. If the atmosphere is hostile it's troublesome.

Nurse Fernando Bustos: I'd inspire you with confidence. I'd show you the pavilion and the equipment for work, and I'd tell you some things about the management of patients. I'd let you know the preferences of the doctors and I'd give you some advice about the attendants. I'd help you in everything possible. I think that's enough.

Nurse Santiago Cruz: First, I'd tell you, well, be a little careful and don't have too much confidence in the patients, because from one minute to another they can react against you. If you have some problem with other professionals, don't feel bad because it happens everywhere, and if there's a disagreement with another nurse you need to know how to bear it. Then I'd explain the methods of working, the schedule, where the equipment is, what's lacking for performing like a nurse, since this is a hospital that lacks equipment, and not to leave for that reason. I'd refer to the personnel and tell you always to have consideration for them in any difficult situation, and to ask for their cooperation and help, and to lend yours as much as you can.

Nurse Ricardo Chivas: The students are getting accustomed to the services, like the young man who just left here. So when you graduate and you have your service you'll already be used to it. The disciplinary part is a little uncomfortable or difficult. You have to know how to understand patients and know how to deal with them. A great deal depends on that. And you need to know how to guide them and lead them, to let them know their obligations to the personnel and to know how to get along with other patients. We have to treat them with respect. You have to have a little confidence with patients--not a lot but a little.

Nurse Sara Delgado: First, not to show fear in front of the patients, but show confidence to them. But you always need to take precautions without showing it. You need to capture the sympathy of the patients and the personnel, and you need to know how to impose your will, but smoothly so that they don't notice. And you need to ask for cooperation from the patients and the personnel very carefully, so that you don't give orders roughly but that you be a little psychological, and that you don't treat them severely but in a friendly way.

Nurse Miguel Esquivel: The advice I always give is to have a great desire to cooperate with the head nurse. Then, not to complain about your lack of experience but to ask the head for his advice, because he will be obliged to give it. The book of experience has no page limit.

Nurse Rosa Frías: I'd tell you it's pleasant and that you're going to get used to it, that life is very good here and that we all have our problems but they all disappear. You need to make friends and take advantage of all the good things here.

Nurse Amada Godoy: At the start, observation of the way the service operates, the management of the pavilion. And I'd explain the way in which each doctor works. I'd tell you about each patient and her clinical history. You'd need to know about their reactions and their treatment so that you can give correct information to the doctor. I'd tell you to be affectionate and kind so they'd accept you and not reject you. I'd also explain to you how to act with the subordinate personnel if there are problems with them.

Nurse Juan Hurtado: In the first place, to be in control of the situation, always be on the alert when you're in a pavilion like this one. Don't trust the patients and take precautions like a new person. And then, be sure of yourself in all your motions and acts with the patients, because sometimes they haven't lost all contact and they notice what's happening. Don't lose your self-assurance.

Nurse María Iglesias: Have patience and take charge of the situation.

Nurse Teodora Justo: Have good will, be serious and responsible in all your actions.

Nurse Héctor Lozada: I'd tell you to look for experience and have self-control.

Nurse Antonio Llona: You have to treat people with regard.

Being a nurse in the Hospital Víctor Larco Herrera has its drawbacks, although some pavilions are more pleasant than others. Our subjects have not lost their devotion to patient care, perhaps the most meaningful symbol of nursing which is instilled in them during their training, but they appear to be overwhelmed by an atmosphere of scarcity, Hospital politics, subordination to doctors, the management of attendants, and hostility on the part of many patients. The central problem for the nurse is to find ways to maximize the exercise of his or her authority in such a way that patients cooperate in their treatment, they are properly fed and clothed, and attendants keep them and the pavilion clean, with everything in place. What lies beneath all of this is the issue of restraint--which, I think, needs to be treated objectively as neither good nor bad in itself but simply as a fact of existence which is to be evaluated only in terms of its *effects* on social actors. This would continue to apply now, as much as it did thirty years ago, when chemical restraint has so sweepingly and ineluctably replaced most forms of physical restraint, which these days take their place as ancient relics in our "museums of madness," the title Scull (1979) chose for his influential book. However, what May (1965:266) observed in those earlier times is still relevant, albeit in a rather different context since times have changed, to contemporary psychiatric nursing and, consequently, psychiatric practice:

> Experience suggests that forms of restraint, however disguised, detract from nurse-patient relationship, interfere with progressive treatment policies, and indirectly contribute to the shortage of nursing staff in hospitals, since "nursing" is replaced by surveillance and control. . . . In some circumstances, control of anti-social behavior is necessary in the patient's interest as well as in that of the hospital community. But though we may wish to limit this approach to specific situations, we cannot expect the nurse to forsake the support of authoritarian discipline in her [sic] dealings with patients unless we substitute some other frame of reference in which she can work.

Such a new frame of reference is not easily to be found for nursing. And, it may be emphasized, these nursing prospects are quite independent of what physicians want or do not want. In large part, the search for such identity will continue to be problematic as long as nursing itself remains uncertain of itself and subordinate. With regard to the uncertainty, Strauss (1966:102) says:

> The position of nursing is particularly interesting for several reasons. To begin with, the nurses successfully laid claim to professional title before most other groups appeared on the medical scene . . . . Yet physicians have never given nurses anything like equal status, and unquestionably many have doubted whether nursing was a genuine profession, rather than merely an assisting occupation, and of rather low order albeit necessary. Nurses themselves reflect some confusion as to whether nursing "really" is a profession.

And with regard to the subordination, May (1965:266) points out: "The traditions of nursing have always tended to place the doctor in an authoritarian position, as the arbiter of treatment and the director of clinical policy." Strauss (1966:62) calls nursing an "embedded" occupation "within a hierarchy of authority," in that "nurses tend to *look upward to physicians* for orders and *downward to assistants* . . . for response to their own orders." Olesen and Whittaker (1968:73) speak of "traditional structures frozen to encapsulate the nurse in a lowly position, not only because of her education, but also because of her femininity." Indeed, Mauksch (1966:131, note 21) raises the intriguing question of what would be "the consequences for the social structure of a hospital if all of its physicians were female and all the nurses were male."

Sensitivity to this status among Peruvian nurses does not appear in interview materials from female nurses but in the responses of some of the male nurses: not only in the resentment expressed by one subject of the use of feminine gender on his certificate but, as well, in other responses which appear to reflect the displacement of feelings into "favoritism" displayed in regard to female nurses.

All of this tends to place nursing in the position of a "second-best" or "second-choice" occupation, despite attempts by nurses to professionalize themselves further. The conflict evident in so many of the interview protocols is impressive; and it is possible that the silence in those where status conflict is not evident may cover deeper conflicts that are not allowed to come to the surface. If it is possible to generalize this to the many nurses in the Hospital who did not speak with me, and possibly even to the Peruvian nursing profession, then it is apparent that nurses were not content to be what they are, or be where they are. While some said that they always wanted to be nurses, that nursing was a vocation for themselves, others wanted to be: an engineer, a policeman, a veterinarian, a midwife, a physician, a dentist, a small businessman, an educational philosopher, and, for a friend of one of them, a priest. One "fell into nursing," trapped by the 1930 "revolution" (which actually marked a transition from one repressive, dictatorial regime to another). Another was a nurse "by chance." And another insisted that "habit becomes liking." Some were awaiting retirement in order to take up some occupation outside nursing. And others spoke frankly of the necessity of doing *something* in order to make a living for themselves, although a number of them complained about inadequate remuneration and the need to work two shifts. Most of them seem to have made a permanent or temporary reconciliation with the realities of their careers. One called himself a "combat soldier," and confronted his displeasure with the idea of "will power." Another declaimed that "it's no use to dream of something else." Thus, a surprising number of the nurses defined their identities in a negative way, in terms of what they were not, in terms of their exclusion.[7]

Meanwhile, the nurses wished to confirm and reconfirm their conceptions of themselves as professionals. They were enthusiastic about learning any technique or method that would place them closer to the physicians: diagnosis, injection, electro-convulsive therapy, or insulin treatment, and thus aid themselves in amplifying their professional identity; and most wished to avoid the fate of being assigned to a service where they could not develop themselves. Although they *called* nursing a profession, in reality they were not certain of that; and so, it turned out, they were not certain of who they were. Thus, while they said that a nurse has to do everything, they wanted to be specialists. And they recognized a need for better instruction in professional skills that would distance them even farther from the attendants. They looked for opportunities to read books, to specialize themselves at greater depth, to be with the physicians and learn from them, to develop administrative tasks, and to control attendants by way of affirming their status as superiors.

How did they face their subordination to physicians, their exclusion from grace, their abandonment by fate? It appears that on the surface they accepted it, or resigned themselves to it, or allowed themselves to be conquered by it. Immediately below this level of discourse there seems only to have been silence. But one can project into their responses a deeper level of feeling, one that reacted to the structural facts of their secondary ranking--secondary, of course, in a social system where there are multiple ranks--and prospects of remaining there always, and one that emitted continuing rage, pain, and longing. Although what Leininger (1970:155) says about hospital dysfunctions is meant to apply to patients, it can also be applied to *all* categories of hospital populations:

> In any system, one can identify *eufunctions* and *dysfunctions* of a system, which may be either intended or unintended, and either explicit or implicit. A hospital system may be viewed as eufunctional since it helps people retain their health status. It is dysfunctional when it seldom helps people get well and stay well. A hospital could also be viewed as dysfunctional when one finds disturbed and dissatisfied people functioning in the system over an extended period of time.

If this statement applies to nurses, and I have no doubt that it does, how are "disturbed and dissatisfied" nurses going to perform eufunctionally? What is urgent is a professional restructuring in order to change conditions, so that nurses (and others) can function therapeutically. Irving (1983:99) gives a definition of psychiatric nursing in which healthy psyches are strategic:

> The effectiveness of the nurse's therapy depends upon her ability to correctly observe, evaluate, and respond to the patient's needs, and that ability is, in turn, directly dependent upon her knowledge, understanding, and skill in interpersonal relations.
>
> All of these statements about psychiatric nursing imply the nurse's therapeutic use of herself in her relationship with the patient. The nurse uses her own healthy personality and the various methods of communication as treatment tools to help the patient make the necessary corrections in his own faulty communication process.

Even more directly, Peplau (1966:132-133) says:

> A psychiatric nurse is first of all an expert clinician. She may also be a teacher, supervisor, administrator, consultant, or researcher, but underlying all these functional positions there should be advanced clinical training. Such clinical expertness revolves around the field's unique aspect or emphasis, in this case, the role of counselor or psychotherapist. . . . The emphasis in psychiatric nursing is *not* on the mother-surrogate role. . . . The emphasis in psychiatric nursing is *not* on the technical subrole. . . . Other nurses in the past and present have believed that technical expertness in giving tubs, packs, coma insulin and care in the pre- and post-phases of electroconvulsive therapy or lobotomy would lead to solutions to mental illness. Technical expertness in giving medication or carrying out procedures associated with nursing is, in my opinion, not the desirable emphasis in psychiatric nursing.

The realization of this new kind of psychiatric nursing involves, as Leininger (1973:10) notes, a change "from the past maintenance of a role predominantly dependent upon and subordinate to the physician to the present self-directed and colleague-sharing role." But this most certainly was not the case in the Peruvian Hospital. Here we confront a rather large contradiction: that people who are dissatisfied with their identity are placed in circumstances where their actions will have great therapeutic impact on the psyches of psychiatric patients, many of whom do not themselves feel comfortable with their identities. This does not necessarily herald a therapeutic disaster, since this seems to be the human condition in many kinds of institutional settings, e.g., schools, churches, military units, government, and so forth. Peruvian psychiatric patients, many of them, get well and go home to love, play, and work. However, it may suggest that more effective therapy could be delivered by happier health professionals. It also suggests, in relation to Peruvian nurses, that the existing structure of nursing, nursing education, the conditions of nurses' employment, their remuneration, expectations, status, and role will all have to disappear and be replaced by something that provides greater satisfaction of their human needs. Until such a restructuring occurs, it is quite possible that a more effective psychotherapy cannot be carried out, or even developed.

Appendix: The Question Schedule for Nurses

1. Name, age, date of interview.
2. Place of birth. Years in Lima.
3. Education. Where?
4. Occupations before becoming a nurse.
5. When did you graduate in nursing? In what school?
6. Why did you choose the occupation of a nurse?
7. How did you get your job in this Hospital?
8. How long have you worked here? Other hospitals or clinics?
9. What do your relatives, your friends, think of your job here?
10. Your salary here?
11. Do you work outside? What work? Salary?
12. Are you married? Children?
13. Is your income sufficient?
14. How long do you plan to continue work here?
15. Do you want to continue in your occpation all your life? If not, what would you like to do?
16. Do you want to continue in psychiatric nursing?
17. How is the job of nurse here in general?
18. In which pavilions have you worked?
19. Which do you prefer? Why?
20. Which don't you like? Why?
21. What schedule have you worked? What do you prefer?
22. What qualifications should a person have to be a nurse?
23. What qualifications should a person have to work as a nurse here?
24. What are the nurse's tasks?
25. Which do you like more? Less?
26. Have you received any special training to carry out the the work of a psychiatric nurse?
27. Are you satisfied with the training? If not, what would you have liked? Should there be special training?
28. Who gives orders to the nurse?

29. How can a nurse be discharged from the job. Why?*
30. Are you at all worried about the possibilities of personal harm?*
31. How do you get a patient up who doesn't want to get up?*
32. How do you make a patient eat who doesn't want to eat?*
33. What do you do when a disturbed patient grabs you?*
34. Should the nurse use force on patients?*
35. What importance does the nurse have in the Hospital?**
36. What is the best aspect of the job? The worst? What advantages does it have?
37. How are the doctors? How do they treat you?**
38. How should the doctor be? What is his duty?**
39. Who is the best doctor in the pavilion? How are the others?
40. How are the attendants?**
41. How should the attendant be?**
42. Whom do you like most in this pavilion? Least?**
43. What type of patient do you like most? Why? Whom do you like in this pavilion?
44. What type of patient do you like least? Why? Whom in this pavilion?
45. What is the nurse's greatest duty? The attendant's? The patient's?**
46. What thing ought Pavilion [n] achieve? What is the goal? Why does it exist?*
47. What thing ought the Hospital Víctor Larco Herrera achieve? What is the goal? Why does it exist?
48. If you could change something in Pavilion [n], what thing or things would they be?
49. What is a mental illness?***
50. Have your ideas changed after working here?
51. What is a hospital like the Hospital Víctor Larco Herrera?*
52. Have your ideas changed after working here?
53. What happened to you when you came to the Hospital to work the first time?
54. What things do you think are most important for getting used to it?
55. What were your greatest difficulties?
56. Suppose that I were a new nurse who had just come into the job, what advice would you give me for getting used to it more rapidly?

* Some of the responses to these questions are given in Chapter 3.
** Some of the responses to these questions are given in Chapter 5.
*** The responses to this question are given in Chapter 2.

Notes

1. I would like here to express my thanks to Javier Mariátegui and the anonymous interviewer: to him for his kindness in locating a social worker who was willing to take on extra work, receiving the interview protocols, and sending them to me; and to her for carrying out a labor which has been thankless until now, and for continuing to be, not nameless, but unnamed.

2. The question schedule I used appears in the Appendix.

3. I employ a similar set of pseudonyms here, as with the Attendants in Chapter 6, giving the nurses first names so that gender may be distinguished.

4. Glaser (ibid.) adds: "A few leaders of American professional nursing have urged nursing to give these tasks back to the doctors so that nurses can concentrate on their own special functions. But their intentions run counter to the sociological axiom that every occupation in achievement-centered societies tries to enhance its public image and self-image, and a common method is to acquire prestigious tasks from a previously more respected occupation. Since they are located in postbasic departments of nursing and in other nonclinical settings, the exponents of independence cannot control the work of the bulk of nurses, who are hospital and outpatient practitioners. Therefore in an entirely unplanned and informal way, the rank and file subverts these leaders' aims by taking prestige where it is most obviously and easily gotten, namely from the technical and life-and-death tasks that are most highly admired by their co-workers and the public."

5. See note 2.

6. While this last statement may seem strange to some readers, in Peruvian popular disease etiology a strong blow on the back can cause tuberculosis. According to Valdivia Ponce and Zapata Agurto (1962:81), 12 subjects out of a sample of 100 male neurotic patients in the Psychiatric Service, Hospital Obrero, responded to a questionnaire to that effect.

7. Sagasti and Hernández (1994:30) make this acute observation of Peruvian character: "*[I]dentities are constructed in a negative way*: because of *not* being this or that: because of *not* having done one thing or another. Positive referents for the construction of identities at the individual, group, organization, or insuitution level are very scarce, abstract, remote, and difficult to link to daily life. The lack of positive referents to identify with makes it difficult to engage with others in the pursuit of common objectives, reinforces the tendencies toward defining oneself by exclusion, and leads to a general loss of values."

Postface

This book has no "Preface" for me to introduce and talk about the text. Because this is being written *afterward*, and not before the text of this book, to call it a "pre-face" would be a significant distortion. Derrida (1981:7) says:

> The preface would announce in the future tense ("this is what you are going to read") the conceptual content or significance (here, that strange strategy without finality, the debility or failure that organizes the *telos* or the *eschaton*, which reinscribes restricted economy within general economy) of what will *already* have been *written*. And thus sufficiently *read* to be gathered up in its semantic tenor and proposed in advance. From the viewpoint of the fore-word, which recreates an intention-to-say after the fact, the text exists as something written--a past--which, under the false appearance of a present, a hidden omnipotent author (in full mastery of his product) is presenting to the reader as his future. Here is what I wrote, then read, and what I am writing that you are going to read. After which you will again be able to take possession of this preface which in sum you have not yet begun to read, even though, once having read it, you will already have anticipated everything that follows and thus you might just as well dispense with reading the rest. The *pre* of the preface makes the future present, represents it, draws it closer, breathes it in, and in going ahead of it puts it ahead. The *pre* reduces the future to the form of manifest presence.

What Derrida is complaining about suggests an initial (final) deconstruction of time in this book, since the aim of the seven Chapters moves toward an ending which, after exploring or inspecting some facets of existence in the Hospital Víctor Larco Herrera, demands a reconstruction of the practice of medical psychology in Peru (and with it a reconstruction of Peruvian society, for neither can be reconstructed without the other), as it existed in 1959, the time of the research which is reported here. But do these chapters mean 1959, or 1995, or 2000 (to pick arbitrarily some future date)? Or do they mean some indeterminate and timeless process which is not-past, not-present, and not- future? It is this kind of "inspection," and no other, that I find myself making, although, to be as honest as I can, that was not my intention in the beginning.

By "inspection" I mean that I endeavored to function as a "consultation anthropologist" (see Stein 1993a) and, after having engaged in an anthropological examination of the Hospital, I now report back to the personnel who were kind enough to receive me and open themselves to me then, in 1959. The term "inspection" is inspired by an article by Bowen (1965:17), entitled "Need for inspection (or survey) of psychiatric hospital services," in which the author, a British psychiatrist, explains his usage:

> I am aware that the very word "inspection" might be thought by some people to carry certain overtones of authority, even perhaps of military authority. Those who feel in this way will recognize that to be a psychiatrist is no guarantee that we have all of us worked out our oedipal difficulties. The word "inspection," however, has about it another and perhaps more acceptable meaning; that is, as one of the classical methods of medical examination. This is particularly applicable to our current difficulties, because the sort of problem with which we are faced in our hospitals can be very much a clinical psychiatric problem. [A survey of psychiatric services in one part of Britain] left me, after the initial shock, with the impression that the difficulties which were encountered were due to inter-personal relationships at least as much as they were due to obvious material shortcomings. The techniques which seemed to me at that time to be applicable were those of psychiatric diagnosis. This implied, amongst other methods of examination, inspection; and the cure seemed to be to formulate both a diagnosis and a rational scheme of treatment.

It would be a most tragic underachievement if an anthropologist assumed a godlike pose and merely inspected a hospital "from the outside," that is, objectively in the sense of being unattached to the object. This is far ("far" implies distance, rather than a negation of distance) from what has been my experience, although in the beginning I believed I was detached (omnipotent?) and could make an inspection objectively. It is, therefore, relevant to commence (to commence this post-face and, thus, to end the book) with an attempt to act out on a word processor Miller's (1990a:147) question: "How does one arrive somewhere when, without knowing it, one has always been there?" Thus, it is useful to me, and I hope it will be to the reader, to relate something more subjective on how the Hospital and I got closer to each other and became attached. Thus, the year, 1959, has less to do with it than I originally thought, and I have less of a craving to defend the age of these materials. Moreover, we may regard anthropology, as Birley (1990:1) regards psychiatry, as an art; and "time is of little or no relevance to the artist." However, the artist is overdetermined so history is indispensable.

I have explained some of the processes involved in the thirty-year preparation of this report in an article on the "hoarding habit" (Stein 1993a), and this need not be repeated here. But I would like, more simply, to tell how these seven chapters were written. The first essay, on Peruvian psychiatrists, was completed in early 1989 in response to an invitation by Renato Alarcón to contribute something to a volume he was editing as a tribute to Javier Mariátegui. Since Dr. Mariátegui had, during the thirty-five years of our friendship, expressed to me many times his eagerness to read the results of my 1959 research on the Hospital, I thought I would try to put together some materials that would reflect the condition of Peruvian psychiatrists. In November, 1988, I climbed up to the top of a cabinet in my office and brought down the dusty box in which my notes had been reposing for so many years; and I went to work in December of the same year, on an article that proved to be amazingly (to me) easy to write. Amazing, because I had experienced so many difficulties, hesitations, and self-doubts in working with the data in the years immediately following the research. The three articles I had produced (Stein 1963, Stein and Oetting 1964, Oetting and Stein 1966), two of them written jointly with a colleague in clinical psychology, were created at as great a distance as I could possibly place between the data and myself. They were extremely difficult for me to construct: emotionally, since I feared succeeding (putting myself on paper for you, reader, to see) even more than I feared failing; and professionally, since I had done no reading on the practice of hospital psychiatry. But, meanwhile, I had discovered that I could read and write. And when I turned back to the Hospital materials, I found them accessible. It was gratifying to discover that I could get closer to them, and I did. I have added some additional illustrative material to the chapter, and so it is somewhat different from the original form of the article, but I believe it retains most of the original "Whiggist" perspective, a feeling and flavor from the time of its writing. I use this term in Porter and Micale's (1994:6) sense of "Whiggism" as "presentist, progressivist, and tenaciously internalist."

In retrospect, therefore, I feel that I was still not close enough to the material for, in accepting psychiatric authority as "natural," I was overlooking medical grandiosity in the form of the biomedical bias which, Kleinman (1980:56-57) notes, views "all of health care through the cognitive framework of [the medical] profession":

> It is amazing to see how intensely this professional ideology is held by otherwise sensitive and responsible health professionals. It is maintained with blind conviction even in the face of evidence to the contrary. Other components of this professional ideology are such commonly encountered dogmas as: Any health-related activities undertaken by patients themselves or by members of the other sectors of the system are dangerous and should not be tolerated. The biological aspects of medical problems are the "real" ones, while the psychosocial and cultural aspects are second order phenomena and are thus less "real" and important. The encounter between doctors and patients (and families) is one between experts and those who are ignorant, so that the doctor's role is to "tell" or give orders to patients, and the patient's role is to listen passively and comply.

While psychiatric specialists would largely (but not completely) have to occupy a much less grandiose prominence than, say, surgeons or internists, there is something about what Goldstein (1987:132-133) calls "the somewhat magical, authoritarian component" of "moral treatment," a "healing power residing in the person of the physician--the so-called enchantment of medical authority," which is instilled during medical-psychiatric training and reinforced by other hospital population categories. Here is how the well-known nineteenth century French psychiatrist Quirol (quoted in Goldstein, ibid.) described it:

> The physician must be, in some manner, the vital principle of a lunatic hospital. It is he who should set everything in motion; he should regularize all actions, just as he has been called upon to be the regulator of all thoughts. . . . The action of the administration, which governs the material aspect of the establishment and supervises all the employees, ought to be hidden. Never should the administration appeal a decision made by the physician, never should it interpose itself between the physician and the lunatics or between the physician and the mon-medical staff. . . . The physician should be invested with an authority from which no one is exempt.

This is, of course, one basis of Dr. Lleras's complaint about the administration of the Peruvian Hospital; and it is appropriate to add that his complaint, being overdetermined, was also quite legitimate.

But to explain the structure in terms of medical grandiosity does not do justice to an on-going hospital process in which medical hegemony is believed to be legitimate by *everyone.* Thus, Caudill, et al. (1952:320), observed that the patients on a North American psychiatric ward "felt that they had to hold to the belief that one's doctor was competent in his therapeutic capacity; one must cooperate with him in order to make any progress and should not question his authority." Similarly, in a study of the expectations patients have of each other in an in-patient psychiatric service of a North American general hospital, Smith and Thrasher (1968:317) state:

> Towards his therapist, the patient is expected to have an attitude of complete faith, confidence, trust and reliance. The stated or assumed wishes of the therapist are taken as the primary guide for the behavior of the patient and no criticism of the therapist is permitted within the context of the larger society. Refusal to see the therapist evokes the strongest of negative sanctions, and any expression of doubt or dislike elicits a strong defence of the therapist from the other patients.

How healthy does a doctor's countertransference have to be to overcome the structure in which he or she functions? We might be led by such a consideration to suspect that a doctor would have to be affected by some pathology in order see himself or herself as less than godlike. However, this does not seem to be the case. In reporting the results of a questionnaire administered to both patients and doctors, Sobell and Ingalls (1968:328) note that in response to the statement, "The doctor is always right," their subjects produced some impressive results:

"Ninety per cent of the doctors disagreed with this statement, whereas over 50 per cent of medical and psychiatric patients of all types agreed with it." They add, interestingly enough: "Unsolicited comments indicated that many medical respondents did not feel comfortable admitting to an authoritarian kind of role, even though it may be rationally [surely, in the context of the relative rationality of biomedicine] required." The irresistable conclusion is that medical grandiosity is constructed by doctors *and everyone else*.

Chapter 2, on concepts of mental illness, seemed to me to be a second step to take from the beginning I had made with the materials from the psychiatrists. The essay was already in the planning stage when, in September 1989, disaster struck in my family in the form of my wife's catastrophic illness. My stable existence appeared to have been swept away, as if by a tidal wave. One of the major defenses against my sadness at loss, fear of being responsible for my own existence, and rage at abandonment was through the continuation of writing, as if to assert to a most uncertain, unstable, and hostile universe: "See, really, nothing has changed!"

As soon as I had completed the current writing project, a book of essays on Andean economic anthropology, I turned back to the Hospital materials. I wrote on Peruvian mental illness ideology, with the assistance of the few sources I possessed in my personal research library, almost as a continuation of work I had done in medical anthropology in rural Peru (Stein 1977, 1981, n.d.) but with information furnished by the several categories of the Hospital population. The chapter was written in February, 1990. I have preserved the basic form of this essay, but I have added some new quotations and citations by way of bringing it somewhat up to date with my reading.

While this second essay was being prepared, the few sources I had available on Peruvian social psychiatry stimulated my appetite to read on psychiatric practice, psychiatric hospital studies, and psychiatric ideology. Since Freud is such a strategic figure, both for those psychiatrists who accept his theoretical and methodological point of view and for those who do not, it seemed to me that I could learn and understand something more about this medical specialty by reading the "Standard Edition" of his psychological works from cover to cover, which I did in 1990 and 1991. I think the experience restructured my thought processes irreversibly, and I began to move in some new directions, not simply in the ways I was dealing with personal problems, which were accumulating at a breathtaking rate, but in the ways I was handling what I was writing about. This is easily to be discerned in Chapter 3, an essay which revolves around the theme of defining a "mental hospital" and its "structural ambivalence," which seemed to me to be parallel collectively to the ambivalence which is experienced individually. I completed a first draft in April-May, 1990, reading as fast as I could, as I wrote. By then I had made contact with the radical critiques of the asylum by Foucault, Goffman, and Szasz, and, while I could not return to the safe haven of "Whiggism," I saw no purpose in destroying it. I have added some additional text and references to the Chapter but it remains rather like I conceived it.

I can point out here that "structural ambivalence" is nothing new. It has been with us all along as an unanticipated consequence of the existence of asylums. Scull (1993:90) presents us with a good statement of the motivational confusion of nineteenth century "reformers" of eighteenth century "brutality":

> As the experience of these early county asylums demonstrates, even those most heavily involved in lunacy reform lacked at the outset any clear idea of what sort of institution they ought to set up, how it was to be run, or why it would ameliorate the condition of the insane. Hence the new asylums' tendency to be modelled on the very places the reformers were within a few years to denounce so vehemently. A concern with protecting society from the disorder threatened by the raving; a desire to simplify life for those charged with administering local poorhouses and jails; and an equally unfocused and unsystematic feeling that the insane themselves deserved to be treated in a more "humane" fashion: all these were shared in varying degrees by the earliest reformers. But they did not amount to a coherent alternative vision of what could, and should, be done.
>
> This lack of a plausible alternative conception of how the insane might be managed was a severe handicap to the reformers. They remained trapped within the conventional assumptions of their society, and continued to defer to the "expertise" of the mad-doctors.

Chapter 4, written in October-November, 1990, after time away from classes in the summer months gave me the opportunity for concentrated reading, deals with what it is like to be a mental patient in the Hospital. It seemed to me like a direction in which the third essay had already pointed me. It reflects further attempts at self-analysis, experiencing on-going personal pain, and further reading. Similarly, as with the other parts, I have added a some new materials. The principal achievement of this Chapter was a growing awareness that the ideological gap between elite and majority sectors of the Hospital population was much more complex than I had realized. While "folk" criteria apply to conceptions of mental illness among the patients and attendants, as distinguished from technical criteria among the professional sectors, it became clear that if patients did not grasp psychiatric conceptions of pathology and etiology they held some fairly sophisticated notions of what psychotherapy was about. At the same time, a "cognitive distance" existed between the professionals and the majority sectors. There was room for improvement in communication.

Chapter 5 was again an extension of the work I had been doing on patients to the Hospital as a whole population. I simply kept on writing from November, 1990, to January, 1991, to take in role definitions in the Hospital population. Transference phenomena were occupying my attention because I was struggling to understand just what it was that I had personally lost, and so it was easier to see such processes in the Hospital. Transference and countertransference in psychotherapy have been strategic concepts, the latter, of course, having been studied much less completely than the former; and, certainly, patients' transferences of a family model to psychiatric hospitals have been observed. Observations of psychiatric personnel's transferences (or countertransferences) are rarer. However, my field materials allowed me to extend the idea to the total population as both collective and individual unconscious and preconscious processes. If the family analogy holds up, if patients are assigned the "helpless infant" role, and doctors and nurses are like so many fathers and mothers to them, then the ruling ideology (i.e., the ideology of the ruling sector) has indeed overemphasized the feelings children have for their parents while, as Miller (1984:237) intriguingly comments, "parents' feelings toward their children have scarcely been examined and are hardly ever the subject of research." It is time for the "rulers" to look again at their feelings toward the "ruled."

I left this book project in February, 1991, to write an early version of the "hoarding habit" essay, one which was published in Spanish in Peru (Stein 1993b). I then spent the next year and a half reading, during which time I rewrote this essay several times until it was finally published in a reoriented and expanded English version (Stein 1993a). It was not until September-October, 1992, that I was ready to take up materials dealing with the Hospital's attendants, their aspirations and their fears, which form Chapter 6. And I did not write Chapter 7, on the nurses, until January-February, 1994. It was the last chapter that I resisted writing the most and the one that, in so many ways, gave me the most satisfaction during and after the writing. I came to see the nurses, less as oppressive authorities concerned with the maintenance of order and discipline on their services, and more as victims of an oppressive social structure. And, in retrospect, those nurses I interviewed were not as silent as I believed while I was writing the chapter; they told me much about their condition.

It has been difficult for Peruvian nurses to envision themselves as doctors' colleagues rather than doctors' orders-takers. Both the strivings and the limits are to be observed in an article by Sánchez de Celli, et al. (1971:220-221), in which these authors offer a redefinition of the nurse's role after the establishment of a "therapeutic community" where the nurses intervene directly in the patient group and "participate playing a much more active and different role" as therapists "integrated into a team." However, they add:

> Nevertheless, their activity distinguishes them from the rest of the team in that their intervention with patients is much more frequent and direct. Psychiatric nursing remains the great part of their daily labor with patients. This fact makes their role much more delicate insofar as their image can be turned into an object of transference or substitution. . . . Transferentially, patients in general see a mother in the nurse. This causes her to have to maintain a therapeutic attitude . . . in view of the emergence of transferential content from the patients. She offers in this way, as far as possible, corrective emotional experiences for precisely those emotional difficulties arising from a conflictive relationship to that image. . . . At other times patients displace reactions to conflictive relations with their therapists toward the nurse and this should also be an object of special concern and observation.

Since the nurse makes decisions "according to commands received in relation to doing therapy from the doctor," we may conclude that the more things change the more constant they remain. It would appear that more sacrifices will be asked of the nurses. In this regard, Miller's (1990b:143) metaphor, based on Rembrandt's well known painting, of Abraham's intended sacrifice of Isaac offers hope:

> If we love life more than obedience and are not prepared to die in the name of obedience and our fathers' lack of critical judgment, then we can no longer wait like Isaac, with our eyes bound and our hands tied, for our fathers to carry out the will of their fathers. . . . But what would happen if Isaac, instead of reaching for the knife, were to use every ounce of his strength to free his hands so that he could remove Abraham's hand from his face? That would change his situation altogether. He would no longer lie there like a sacrificial lamb but would stand up; he would dare to use his eyes and see his father as he really is: uncertain and hesitant yet intent on carrying out a command he does not comprehend.

It is not too much to ask the people of any hospital to be more aware of who they are and what they are trying to do. Internal awareness, it seems to me, as much of it as possible, ought to be a precondition for any reform effort (as well as any revolution!). But an awareness of external structures and processes must accompany it. Freud (1955b:305) defined the limits of his method in a classic statement at the end of *Studies on Hysteria* in 1895:[1]

> When I have promised my patients help or improvement by means of a cathartic treatment I have often been faced by this objection: "Why, you tell me yourself that my illness is probably connected with my circumstances and the events of my life. You cannot alter these in any way. How do you propose to help me, then?" And I have been able to make this reply: "No doubt fate would find it easier than I do to relieve you of your illness. But you will be able to convince yourself that much will be gained if we succeed in transforming your hysterical misery into common unhappiness. With a mental life that has been restored to health you will be better armed against that unhappiness.

"Hysterial misery" or "common unhappiness?" A choice, of course, but one which leaves much to be desired. It should be pointed out that the condition of the Hospital Víctor Larco Herrera was in 1959 and is at present overdetermined. A more effective understanding of its internal structure by its population would hardly address the issues of the poverty of the country, the indifference of its rulers, and the greed of those who extract its wealth. The external structure weighs heavily on the Hospital and its population. Consequently, we may not call on it "to get its act together," because much has to change in Peru as a whole, and in the world, before we can expect a resolution of its structural ambivalence.

Amherst, New York
June 12, 1995.

Note

1. I am indebted to Masson (1991:207-209) for his exploration of the significance of this passage from Freud.

Bibliography

Alarcón, Renato D. 1990. *Identidad de la psiquiatría latinoamericana, voces y exploraciones en torno a una ciencia solidaria.* México: Siglo Veintiuno Editores.

Allderidge, Patricia. 1985. Bedlam: fact or fantasy? In *The Anatomy of Madness, Essays in the History of Psychiatry, Volume II, Institutions and Society*, W. F. Bynum, Roy Porter, and Michael Shepherd, eds. London and New York: Tavistock Publications.

Arnillas Arana, J. Max, Próspero Otárola T., and collaborators. 1970. Una experiencia de comunidad terapéutica en el Pabellón No. 6 del Hospital "Víctor Larco Herrera". In *Psiquiatría peruana, Primer Congreso Nacional de Psiquiatría*, Oscar Valdivia Ponce y Alberto Péndola Febres, eds. Lima: Editorial Imprenta "Amauta."

Barton, Russell. 1966. *Institutional Neurosis.* Bristol, England: John Wright and Sons.

Bechtel, Robert B., y Alvaro González. 1986. Comparación de ambientes de tratamiento entre algunos hospitales mentales peruanos y norteamericanos. In *Psicología y realidad peruana, el aporte objetivo*, Federico R. León, ed. Lima: Mosca Azul Editores.

Belknap, Ivan. 1956. *Human Problems of a State Mental Hospital.* New York: McGraw-Hill Book Company.

Bellaby, Paul, and Patrick Oribabor. 1980. 'The history of the present'--contradiction and struggle in nursing. In *Rewriting Nursing History*, Celia Davies, ed. London and Totowa, New Jersey: Croom Helm and Barnes & Noble Books.

Birley, James. 1990. The history of psychiatry as the history of an art. In psychiatry as the history of an art. In *Lectures on the History of Psychiatry*, R. M. Murray and T. H. Turner, eds. London: Gaskell.

Bockoven, J. Sanbourne. 1972. *Moral Treatment in Community Mental Health.* New York: Springer Publishing Company.

Bowen, W. A. L. 1965. Need for inspection (or survey) of psychiatric hospital services. In *Psychiatric Hospital Care, a Symposium*, Hugh Freeman, ed. London: Baillière, Tindall & Cassell.

Braginsky, Benjamin M., Dorothea D. Braginsky, and Kenneth Ring. 1969. *Methods of Madness, the Mental Hospital as a Last Resort.* New York: Holt, Rinehart and Winston.

Burnham, Donald L., Arthur I. Gladstone, and Robert W. Gibson. 1969. *Schizophrenia and the Need-Fear Dilemma.* New York: International Universities Press.

Castel, Robert, Francoise Castel, and Anne Lovell. 1982. *The Psychiatric Society.* Translated by Arthur Goldhammer. New York: Columbia University Press.

Caudill, William. 1958. *The Psychiatric Hospital As a Small Society.* Cambridge, Massachusetts: Harvard University Press.

_____, Fredrick C Redlich, Helen R. Gilmore, and Eugene B. Brody. 1952. Social structure and interaction processes on a psychiatric ward. *American Journal of Orthopsychiatry* 22:314-334.

Chamberlin, Judi. 1978. *On Our Own, Patient-Controlled Alternatives to the Mental Health System.* New York: Hawthorn Books.

Chiappe Costa, Mario. 1979. Nosografía curanderil. In *Psiquiatría folklórica, shamanes y curanderos*, Carlos Alberto Seguín, ed. Lima: Ediciones Ermar.

_____, Moisés Lemlij, and Luis Millones. 1985. *Alucinógenos y shamanismo en el Perú contemporáneo.* Lima: Ediciones El Virrey.

Colarelli, Nick J., and Saul M. Siegel. 1966. *Ward H. an Adventure in Innovation.* Princeton, New Jersey: D. Van Nostrand

Company.

Conn, Louis M., and John R. Lion. 1983. Assaults in a university hospital. In *Assaults within Psychiatric Facilities*, John R. Lion and William H. Reid, eds. New York and London: Grune and Stratton.

Cooper, David. 1967. *Psychiatry and Anti-Psychiatry*. London: Tavistock Publications.

Coser, Ruth Laub. 1962. *Life in the Ward*. East Lansing, Michigan: Michigan State University Press.

Custred, Glynn. 1979. Inca concepts of soul and spirit. In *Essays in Humanistic Anthropology: a* Festschrift *in Honor of David Bidney*. Washington: University Press of America.

Dain, Norman. 1964. *Concepts of Insanity in the United States, 1789-1865*. New Brunswick, New Jersey: Rutgers University Press.

Delgado, Honorio. 1989. *Freud y el psicoanálisis, escritos y testimonio*. Lima: Universidad Peruana Cayetano Heredia, Fondo Editorial.

_____ 1992. *Honorio Delgado en* El Comercio. Lima: Ediciόn de "El Comercio."

Derrida, Jacques. 1978. *Writing and Difference*. Translated by Alan Bass. Chicago: The University of Chicago Press.

_____ 1981. *Dissemination*. Translated by Barbara Johnson. Chicago and London: The University of Chicago Press.

Dunham, H. Warren, and S. Kirson Weinberg. 1960. *The Culture of the State Mental Hospital*. Detroit: Wayne State University Press.

Dwyer, Ellen. 1987. *Homes for the Mad, Life Inside Two Nineteenth-Century Asylums*. New Brunswick, New Jersey, and London: Rutgers University Press.

Erikson, Kai T. 1970 [1957]. Patient role and social uncertainty--a dilemma of the mentally ill. In *Social System Perspectives in Residential Institutions*, Howard W. Polsky, Daniel S. Claster and Carl Goldberg, eds. East Lansing, Michigan: Michigan State University Press.

Estroff, Sue E. 1981. *Making It Crazy, an Ethnography of Psychiatric Clients in an American Community*. Berkeley, California: University of California Press.

Etzioni, Amitai. 1970. Interpersonal structural factors in the study of mental hospitals. In *Social System Perspectives in Residential Institutions*, Howard W. Polsky, Daniel S. Claster, and Carl

Goldberg, eds. East Lansing, Michigan: Michigan State University Press.

Falloon, Ian R. H. 1988. Social skills training for schizophrenia. In *The Schizophrenias*, Frederic Flach, ed. New York and London: W. W. Norton and Company.

Foucault, Michel. 1965. *Madness and Civilization, a History of Insanity in the Age of Reform.* Translated from the French by Richard Howard. New York: Pantheon Books.

_____ 1990. *The History of Sexuality. Volume I: an Introduction.* Translated from the French by Robert Hurley. New York: Vintage Books.

Fox, Richard W. 1978. *So Far Disordered in Mind, Insanity in California, 1870-1930.* Berkeley: University of California Press.

Freidson, Eliot. 1970a. *Professional Dominance: the Social Structure of Medical Care.* New York: Atherton Press.

_____ 1970b. *Profession of Medicine, a Study of the Sociology of Applied Knowledge.* New York: Dodd, Mead and Company.

Freud, Anna, and Dorothy T. Burlingham. 1943. *War and Children.* London: Medical War Books.

Freud, Sigmund. 1955a. The "uncanny." In *The Standard Edition of the Complete Psychological Works of Sigmund Freud. Volume XVII (1917-1919).* Translated by James Strachey. London: The Hogarth Press and the Institute of Psycho-analysis.

_____ 1955b. The psychotherapy of hysteria. In Studies on Hysteria by Josef Breuer and Sigmund Freud. In *The Standard Edition of the Complete Psychological Works of Sigmund Freud. Volume II (1893-1895).* Translated by James Strachey. London: The Hogarth Press and the Institute of Psycho-analysis.

Glaser, William A. 1963. American and foreign hospitals: some sociological comparisons. In *The Hospital in Modern Society*, Eliot Freidson, ed. New York: The Free Press of Glencoe.

_____. 1966. Nursing leadership and policy: some cross-national comparisons. In *The Nursing Profession: Five Sociological Essays*, Fred Davis, ed. New York: John Wiley & Sons.

Goffman, Erving. 1962. *Asylums, Essays on the Social Situation of Mental Patients and Other Inmates.* Chicago: Aldine Publishing Company.

Goldstein, Jan. 1987. *Console and Classify, the French Psychiatric Profession in the Nineteenth Century.* Cambridge, England:

Cambridge University Press.

González Uzcátegui, René. 1991. Programación de salud mental en América Latina. In *"Desde nuestra propia entraña," homenaje al Profesor Javier Mariátegui*, Renato D. Alarcón, ed. Lima: Universidad Peruana Cayetano Heredia.

Greenblatt, Milton. 1955. Toward a therapeutic community. In *From Custodial to Therapeutic Patient Care in Mental Hospitals, Explorations in Social Treatment*, Milton Greenblatt, Richard H. York, and Esther Lucile Brown. New York: Russell Sage Foundation.

Grob, Gerald N. 1966. *The State and the Mentally Ill, a History of Worcester State Hospital in Massachusetts, 1830-1920.* Chapel Hill, North Carolina: University of North Carolina Press.

_____ 1973. *Mental Institutions in America, Social Policy to 1875.* New York and London: The Free Press/Collier Macmillan Publishers.

_____ 1979. Rediscovering asylums: the unhistorical history of the mental hospital. In *The Therapeutic Revolution, Essays in the Social History of American Medicine*, Morris J. Vogel and Charles E. Rosenberg, eds. Philadelphia: University of Pennsylvania Press.

_____ 1983. *Mental Illness and American Society, 1875-1940.* Princeton, New Jersey: Princeton University Press.

_____ 1985. *The Inner World of American Psychiatry, 1890-1940, Selected Correspondence.* New Brunswick, New Jersey: Rutgers University Press.

_____ 1991. *From Asylum to Community, Mental Health Policy in Modern America.* Princeton, New Jersey: Princeton University Press.

_____ 1994. The history of asylums revisited: personal reflections. In *Discovering the History of Psychiatry*, Mark S. Micale and Roy Porter, eds. New York: Oxford University Press.

Haugsgjerd, Svein. 1980. Report from Norway. In *Critical Psychiatry, the Politics of Mental Health*, David Ingleby, ed. New York: Pantheon Books.

Henry, Jules. 1954. The formal social structure of a psychiatric hospital. *Psychiatry* 17:139-151.

_____ 1964. Space and power on a psychiatric unit. In *The Psychiatric Hospital as a Social System*, Albert F. Wessen, ed.

Springfield, Illinois: Charles C. Thomas.

Hyde, Robert W. 1955. *Experiencing the Patient's Day*. New York: G. P. Putnam's Sons.

Ingleby, David. 1980. Understanding "mental illness." In *Critical Psychiatry, the politics of mental health*, David Ingleby, ed. New York: Pantheon Books.

Irving, Susan. 1983. *Basic Psychiatric Nursing*. Third edition. Philadelphia: W. B. Saunders Company.

James, F. E. 1992. Insulin treatment in psychiatry. *History of Psychiatry* 3:221-235.

Jones, Kathleen. 1955. *Lunacy, Law, and Conscience, 1744-1845, the Social History of the Care of the Insane*. London: Routledge and Kegan Paul.

_____ 1982 Scull's dilemma. *British Journal of Psychiatry* 141:221-226.

_____ 1991 The culture of the mental hospital. In *150 Years of British Psychiatry, 1841-1991*. London: Gaskell.

Jones, Maxwell. 1953. *The Therapeutic Community, a New Treatment Method in Psychiatry*. New York: Basic Books.

_____ 1962. *Social Psychiatry, in the Community, in Hospitals, and in Prisons*. Springfield, Illinois: Charles C. Thomas Publisher.

_____ 1968 *Beyond the Therapeutic Community, Social Learning and Social Psychiatry*. New Haven, Connecticut, and London: Yale University Press.

Kalkman, Marion E. 1974. Models of psychiatric treatment. In *New Dimensions in Mental Health-Psychiatric Nursing*, Marion E. Kalkman and Anne J. Davis, eds. New York: McGraw-Hill Book Company.

Kiesler, Charles A., and Amy Sibulkin. 1987. *Mental Hospitalization, Myths and Facts about a National Crisis*. Beverly Hills, California: Sage Publications.

Klein, Melanie. 1975. *Envy and Gratitude, and Other Works*. London: The Hogarth Press and the Institute of Psycho-Analysis.

Kleinman, Arthur. 1980. *Patients and Healers in the Context of Culture, an Exploration of the Borderland between Anthropology, Medicine, and Psychiatry*. Berkeley, California: University of California Press.

Kraft, Alan M. 1981. Discussion: systems for the chronically mentally ill. In *The Chronic Mentally Ill, Treatment, Programs,*

Systems. New York: Human Sciences Press.

Kris, Ernst. 1975. *Selected Papers of Ernst Kris*. New Haven, Connecticut: Yale University Press.

Kubie, Lawrence S. 1975. The responsibility of the medical profession to provide hospital treatment. In *The Future Role of the State Hospital*, Jaci Zusman and Elmer F. Bertsch, eds. Lexington, Massachusetts: Lexington Books.

LeBar, Frank M. 1964. Some implications of ward structure for enculturation of patients. In *The Psychiatric Hospital as a Social System*, Albert F. Wessen, ed. Springfield, Illinois: Charles C. Thomas.

Leininger, Madeleine M. 1970. *Nursing and Anthropology: Two Worlds to Blend*. New York: John Wiley & Sons.

_____ 1973. Winds of change. In *Contemporary Issues in Mental Health Nursing*, Madeleine M. Leininger, ed. Boston: Little, Brown and Company.

Levinson, Daniel J., and Eugene B. Gallagher. 1964. *Patienthood in the Mental Hospital, an Analysis of Role, Personality, and Social Structure*. Boston: Houghton Mifflin Company.

Linn, Louis. 1964. Some aspects of a psychiatry program in a voluntary general hospital. In *Handbook of Community Psychiatry and Community Mental Health*, Leopold Bellak, ed. New York and London: Grune and Stratton.

Lion, John R. 1988. The violent patient: assessment and management. In *The Schizophrenias*, Frederic Flach, ed. New York and London: W. W. Norton and Company.

Loeb, Martin B. 1968. Some dominant cultural themes in a psychiatric hospital. In *The Mental Patient, Studies in the Sociology of Deviance*, Stephan P. Spitzer and Norman K. Denzin, eds. New York: McGraw-Hill Book Company.

Luchins, Abraham S. 1959. *A Functional Approach to Training in Clinical Psychology, Via Study of a Mental Hospital*. Springfield, Illinois: Charles C. Thomas.

Luske, Bruce. 1990. *Mirrors of Madness, Patrolling the Psychic Border*. New York: Aldine De Gruyter.

Mariátegui, José Carlos. 1959. *El Alma Matinal y Otras Estaciones del Hombre de Hoy*. Lima: Biblioteca Amauta.

Mariátegui Chiappe, Javier. 1985a. *La psiquiatría peruana en sus figuras representativas*. Lima: Instituto Nacional de Salud Mental

"Honorio Delgado-Hideo Noguchi".

_____ 1985b *Baltazar Caravedo Prado, la generación de 900 y la psiquiatría.* Fascículo editado en adhesión al Homenaje a Baltazar Caravedo y a Víctor Larco Herrera por la Asociación Psiquiátrica Peruana en el Primer Congreso Nor-Peruano y Primer Congreso Peruano-Ecuatoriano de Psiquiatría, Trujillo.

_____ 1987 La psiquiatría y su santoral en el Perú. *Acta Psiquiátrica y Psicológica de América Latina* 33:257-258.

_____ 1988 *Salud mental y realidad nacional, el primer quinquenio del Instituto Nacional de Salud Mental.* Lima: Biblioteca de Psiquiatría Peruana.

_____ 1990 Hermilio Valdizán y la psiquiatría peruana. In *Paleopsiquiatría del antiguo Perú*, Hermilio Valdizán. Lima: Universidad Peruana Cayetano Heredia.

_____, et al. 1966. Ensayo terapéutico con un derivado fenotiacínico de acción prolongada, el enantato de flufenacina en un grupo de esquizofrénicos crónicos. *Revista de Neuro-Psiquiatría* (Lima) 29:33-44.

Martini P., Claudio. 1983. *El fin del manicomio.* México: Ediciones Nueva Sociología.

Masson, Jeffrey Moussaieff. 1991. *Final Analysis, the Making and Unmaking of a Psychoanalyst.* New York: Harper Perennial.

Mauksch, Hans O. 1966. The organizational context of nursing practice. In *The Nursing Profession: Five Sociological Essays*, Fred Davis, ed. New York: John Wiley & Sons.

May, A. R. 1965. Observations on training the psychiatric nurse. In *Psychiatric Hospital Care, a Symposium*, Hugh Freeman, ed. London: Baillière, Tindall & Cassell.

McGovern, Constance M. 1985. *Masters of Madness, Social Origins of the American Psychiatric Profession.* Hanover, New Hampshire: University Press of New England.

Mechanic, David. 1980. *Mental Health and Social Policy.* Second edition. Englewood Cliffs, New Jersey: Prentice-Hall.

Mellett, David J. 1982. *The Prerogative of Asylumdom, Social, Cultural, and Administrative Aspects of the Institutional Treatment of the Insane in Nineteenth-Century Britain.* New York and London: Garland Publishing.

Menzies Lyth, Isabel. 1988. *Containing Anxiety in Institutions, Selected Essays. Volume I.* London: Free Association Books.

Miller, Alice. 1984. *Thou Shalt Not Be Aware, Society's Betrayal of the Child.* Translated by Hildegarde and Hunter Hannum. New York: Farrar, Straus, Giroux.

_____ 1990a *Banished Knowledge, Facing Childhood Injuries.* Translated from the German by Leila Vennewitz. New York: Doubleday.

_____ 1990b *The Untouched Key, Tracing Childhood Trauma in Creativity and Destructiveness.* Translated from the German by Hildegard Hannum and Hunter Hannum. New York: Doubleday.

Moos, Rudolf H. 1974. *Evaluating Treatment Environments, a Social Ecological Approach.* New York: John Wiley and Sons.

Morrissey, Joseph P., Howard H. Goldman, and Lorraine V. Klerman. 1980. Approaches to the study of institutional reform. In *The Enduring Asylum, Cycles of Institutional Reform at Worcester State Hospital*, Joseph P. Morrissey, Howard H. Goldman, and Lorraine V. Klerman, eds. New York: Grune and Stratton.

Naboisek, Herbert, Ozzie G. Simmons, Dorothy M. Mathews and Stanley H. Cath. 1957. Hospital image and post-hospital experience. In *The Patient and the Mental Hospital*, Milton Greenblatt, Daniel J. Levinson and Richard H. Williams, eds. Glencoe, Illinois: The Free Press.

Oetting, E. R., and William W. Stein. 1966. Popular medical beliefs and attitude toward mental illness in Peru. *Human Organization* 25:308-311.

Olesen, Virginia L., and Elvi W. Whittaker. 1968. *The Silent Dialog, a Study in the Social Psychology of Professional Socialization.* San Francisco: Jossey-Bass.

Osborne, Oliver H. 1973. Anthropological issues in mental health nursing. In *Contemporary Issues in Mental Health Nursing*, Madeleine M. Leininger, ed. Boston: Little, Brown and Company.

Parry-Jones, William Ll. 1972. *The Trade in Lunacy, a Study of Private Madhouses in England in the Eighteenth and Nineteenth Centuries.* London and Toronto: Routledge & Kegan Paul, University of Toronto Press.

Parsons, Talcott. 1957. The mental hospital as a type of organization. In *The Patient and the Mental Hospital*, Milton Greenblatt, Daniel J. Levinson and Richard H. Williams, eds. Glencoe, Illinois: The Free Press.

Peplau, Hildegard E. 1966. Interpersonal techniques: the crux of psychiatric nursing. in *Psychiatric Nursing, Developing Psychiatric Nursing Skills*, Dorothy Mereness, ed. Dubuque, Iowa: Wm. C. Brown Company Publishers.

Porter, Roy. 1987a. *Mind-Forg'd Manacles, a History of Madness in England from the Restoration to the Regency*. London: The Athlone Press.

______ 1987b *A Social History of Madness, Stories of the Insane*. London: Weidenfeld and Nicolson.

_____ and Mark S. Micale. 1994. Introduction: reflections on psychiatry and its histories. In *Discovering the History of Psychiatry*, Mark S. Micale and Roy Porter, eds. New York: Oxford University Press.

Rapoport, Robert N. 1960. *Community as Doctor, New Perspectives on a Therapeutic Community*. London and Springfield, Illinois: Tavistock Publications and Charles C. Thomas.

Rhodes, Lorna A. 1991. *Emptying Beds, the Work of an Emergency Psychiatric Unit*. Berkeley, California: University of California Press.

Robinson, Alice M. 1964. *Psychiatric Aide*. Philadelphia: J. P. Lippincott Company.

Romanucci-Ross, Lola. 1983. On madness, deviance, and culture. In *The Anthropology of Medicine, from Culture to Method*, Lola Romanucci-Ross, Daniel E. Moerman, and Laurence R. Tancredi, eds. New York: Praeger.

Rotondo, Humberto. 1960. Explicaciones orales-agresivas de enfermedad en una población mestiza. In *Estudios sobre personalidad básica en mestizos*. Lima: Departamento de Higiene Mental, Ministerio de Salud Pública y Asistencia Social.

Rubenstein, Robert, and Harold D. Lasswell. 1966. *The Sharing of Power in a Psychiatric Hospital*. New Haven, Connecticut, and London: Yale University Press.

Ruiz Zevallos, Augusto. 1994. *Psiquiatrías y locos, entre la modernización contra los Andes y el nuevo proyecto de modernidad, Perú, 1850-1930*. Lima: Instituto Pasado & Presente.

Sagasti, Francisco, and Max Hernández. 1994. The crisis of governance. In *Peru in Crisis: Dictatorship or Democracy?*, Joseph S. Tulchin and Gary Bland, eds. Boulder, Colorado, and

London: Lynne Rienner Publishers.

Salisbury, Richard F. 1962. *Structures of Custodial Care, an Anthropological Study of a State Mental Hospital.* Berkeley, California: University of California Press.

Sánchez de Celli, Nélida, Sara Barboza de Aguilar, Manuel Tantaleán, and Armando Martell. 1971. Rol de la enfermera en la comunidad terapéutica del Hospital Obrero de Lima. In *Anales del Segundo Congreso Nacional de Psiquiatría*, Fernando Samanez Concha, Rubén Ríos Carrasco and Moisés Lemlij Malamud, eds. Lima: Asociación Psiquiátrica Peruana.

Sarwer-Foner, G. J. 1961. Comment. In *Mental Patients in Transition, Steps in Hospital-Community Rehabilitation*, Milton Greenblatt, Daniel J. Levinson and Gerald L. Klerman, eds. Springfield, Illinois: Charles C. Thomas.

Scull, Andrew T. 1977. *Decarceration, Community Treatment and the Deviant: a Radical View.* Englewood Cliffs, New Jersey: Prentice-Hall.

_____ 1979 *Museums of Madness, the Social Organization of Insanity in Nineteenth-Century England.* New York: St. Martin's Press.

_____ 1991 Psychiatry and social control in the nineteenth and twentieth centuries. *History of Psychiatry* 2:149-169.

_____ 1993 *The Most Solitary of Afflictions, Madness and Society in Britain, 1700-1900.* New Haven and London: Yale University Press.

_____, ed. 1981. *Madhouses, Mad-Doctors, and Madmen, the Social History of Psychiatry in the Victorian Era.* Philadelphia: University of Pennsylvania Press.

Sedgwick, Peter. 1982. *Psycho Politics.* New York: Harper and Row.

Seguín, Carlos Alberto. 1979. Introducción a la psiquiatría folklórica. In *Psiquiatría folklórica, shamanes y curanderos*, Carlos Alberto Seguín, ed. Lima: Ediciones Ermar.

Sharkey, Joe. 1994. *Bedlam, Greed, Profiteering, and Fraud in a Mental Health System Gone Crazy.* New York: St. Martin's Press.

Smith, Harvey L., and Daniel J. Levinson. 1957. The major aims and organizational characteristics of mental hospitals. In *The Patient and the Mental Hospital, Contributions of Research in the Science of Social Behavior*, Milton Greenblatt, Daniel J. Levinson and Richard H. Williams, eds. Glencoe, Illinois: The Free Press.

Smith, Harvey L., and Jean Thrasher. 1968. Roles, cliques, and sanctions: dimensions of patient society. In *The Mental Patient, Studies in the Sociology of Deviance*, Stephan P. Spitzer and Norman K. Denzin, eds. New York: McGraw-Hill Book Company.

Snyder, William, III. 1983. Administrative monitoring of assaultive patients and staff. In *Assaults within Psychiatric Facilities*, John R. Lion and William H. Reid, eds. New York and London: Grune and Stratton.

Sobel, Raymond, and Ardis Ingalls. 1968. Resistance to treatment: explorations of the patient's sick role. In *The Mental Patient, Studies in the Sociology of Deviance*, Stephan P. Spitzer and Norman K. Denzin, eds. New York: McGraw-Hill Book Company.

Soloff, Paul H. 1983. Seclusion and restraint. In *Assaults within Psychiatric Facilities*, John R. Lion and William H. Reid, eds. New York and London: Grune and Stratton.

Spiegel, John P. 1957. The resolution of the role conflict within the family. In *The Patient and the Mental Hospital, Contributions of Research in the Science of Social Behavior*, Milton Greenblatt, Daniel J. Levinson, and Richard H. Williams, eds. Glencoe, Illinois: The Free Press.

Stanton, Alfred H., and Morris S. Schwartz. 1954. *The Mental Hospital, a Study of Institutional Participation in Psychiatric Illness and Treatment*. New York: Basic Books.

_____ 1970 The management of a type of institutional participation in mental illness. In *Social System Perspectives in Residential Institutions*, Howard Polsky, Daniel S. Claster and Carl Goldberg, eds. East Lansing, Michigan: Michigan State University Press. [1949.]

Stein, William W. 1963a. Patterns of a Peruvian mental hospital. *International Journal of Social Psychiatry* 10:208-215.

_____ 1963b. Esquema de un hospital mental peruano. *Boletin de la Division de Higiene Mental* 5/6(1), 1963.

_____ 1977. Modernización y retroceso del mito: diagnosis por medio de la magia y curación en el pueblo de Vicos, Perú. *América Indígena* 37:671-647.

_____ 1981. The folk illness: entity or nonentity? An essay on

Vicos disease ideology. In *Health in the Andes*, Joseph W. Bastien and John M. Donahue, eds. Washington: American Anthropological Association.

_____ 1984. How peasants are exploited: the extraction of unpaid labor in rural Peru. In *Research in Economic Anthropology* 6:273-308. Greenwich, Connecticut: JAI Press.

_____ 1993a. The hoarding habit, countertransference, and consultation anthropology in a Peruvian psychiatric hospital. *Social Science and Medicine* 37:1045-1054.

_____ 1993b. El hábito de coleccionismo en un hospital mental peruano. *Revista de Neuro-Psiquiatría* (Lima) 54:40-46.

_____ n.d. Popular Medicine in Peru: Program or Root? Exploring the Infrastructure of Medical Practice. Paper presented to the Congreso Mundial de Medicina Folklórica, Lima, October 26-November 2, 1979.

_____, and E. R. Oetting. 1964. Humanism and custodialism in a Peruvian mental hospital. *Human Organization* 23:278-282.

Strauss, Anselm. 1966. The structure and ideology of American nursing: an interpretation. In *The Nursing Profession: Five Sociological Essays*, Fred Davis, ed. New York: John Wiley & Sons.

_____, Leonard Schatzman, Rue Bucher, Danuta Ehrlich and Melvin Sabshin. 1964. *Psychiatric Ideologies and Institutions*. New York and London: The Free Press of Glencoe/Collier-Macmillan Limited.

_____, Leonard Schatzman, Danuta Ehrlich, Rue Bucher and Melvin Sabshin. 1963. The hospital and its negotiated order. In *The Hospital in Modern Society*, Eliot Freidson, ed. New York: The Free Press of Glencoe.

Szasz, Thomas S. 1970. *The Manufacture of Madness, a Comparative Study of the Inquisition and the Mental Health Movement*. New York: Harper and Row, Publishers.

Talbott, John A. 1978. *The Death of the Asylum, a Critical Study of State Hospital Management, Services, and Care*. New York: Grune and Stratton.

Tomes, Nancy. 1984. *A Generous Confidence, Thomas Story Kirkbride and the Art of Asylum-Keeping, 1840-1883*. Cambridge, England: Cambridge University Press.

Valdivia Ponce, Oscar. 1989. *Panorama de la psiquiatría en el Perú*.

Lima: Universidad Nacional Mayor de San Marcos.

_____ and Sergio Zapata Agurto. 1962. Concepciones sobre medicina popular en pacientes neuróticos. In *Psiquiatría y sociedad, estudios sobre la realidad peruana*, Carlos Alberto Seguín, ed. Lima: Universidad Nacional Mayor de San Marcos.

Valdizán, Hermilio. 1988. *Locos de la colonia.* Lima: Instituto Nacional de Cultura.

Webb, Richard C. 1977. *Government Policy and the Distribution of Income in Peru, 1963-1973.* Cambridge, Massachusetts, and London: Harvard University Press.

Wing, J. K., and G. W. Brown. 1970. *Institutionalism and Schizophrenia, a Comparative Study of Three Mental Hospitals, 1960-1968.* Cambridge, England: Cambridge University Press.

York, Richard H. 1955. Experiments in ward patient care at Bedford Veterans Administration Hospital. In *From Custodial to Therapeutic Patient Care in Mental Hospitals, Explorations in Social Treatment*, Milton Greenblatt, Richard H. York, and Esther Lucile Brown. New York: Russell Sage Foundation.

Index